SELF-ASSESS
THE DIPL.... IN
CHILD HEALTH

Wai-Ching Leung

Senior Registrar in Public Health
Department of Public Health
Sunderland Health Authority
Sunderland, UK

Adrian Minford

Consultant Paediatrician
St Luke's Hospital
Bradford
West Yorkshire, UK

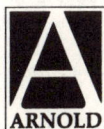

A member of the Hodder Headline Group
LONDON • SYDNEY • AUCKLAND
Co-published in the USA by Oxford University Press, Inc., New York

Arnold, a member of the Hodder Headline Group,
338 Euston Road, London NW1 3BH

Co-published in the United States of America by
Oxford University Press, Inc.,
198 Madison Avenue, New York, NY 10016
Oxford is a registered trademark of Oxford University Press

British Library Cataloguing in Publication Data
A catalogue record for this book is available from the British Library

Library of Congress Cataloging-in-Publication Data
A catalog record for this book is available from the Library of Congress

ISBN 0 340 67720 1(Pb)

Typeset in 10/12pt Helvetica by Gray Publishing, Tunbridge Wells
Printed and bound in Great Britain by J. W. Arrowsmith

CONTENTS

PREFACE

The Diploma in Child Health (DCH) Examination is taken by doctors aiming for a career in general practice and by some paediatric trainees prior to sitting the MRCP (Paediatrics) examination. It is the second most popular postgraduate examination after the DRCOG examination.

There is an abundance of revision books for Parts I and II of the MRCP (Paediatrics) examination. However, there are significant differences in both content and format between the DCH examination and the MRCP (Paediatrics) examination. The latter focuses on childhood diseases and their treatment, whereas the former focuses on child health. Community child health, prevention of childhood disorders, child health surveillance, legislation relating to children, education, social services for children, and emotional development and disorders are important components of the DCH syllabus. The DCH written examination consists of multiple choice questions, short-note questions and case commentaries. This differs substantially from the data interpretation, slides and grey cases of the MRCP (Paediatrics) examination. In the clinical examination, a specific section of the DCH is devoted to developmental assessment and the testing of hearing and vision.

There are, at present, no revision books on the market which specifically target the DCH syllabus both in terms of content and format. The aim of this book is to fill this gap and to allow candidates to have the opportunity to review their examination techniques in all sections of the examination and to practice answering written papers. The Introductory Section gives guidance on the clinical and other sections of the examination. This is followed by five papers, each consisting of multiple choice questions, short note questions and case commentary papers. These are supported by detailed explanations for the multiple choice questions and model answers for the short note and case commentary papers.

We hope that this book will be a useful guide and revision aid for prospective DCH candidates.

Wai-Ching Leung
Adrian Minford

INTRODUCTION

The Diploma in Child Health Examination is suitable for general practitioners or trainees who wish to have recognition of their competence in looking after children. It is well-respected and is usually accepted for accreditation of general practitioners in Child Health Surveillance. The examination is also suitable for paediatric trainees without the necessary experience to sit for the MRCP(UK) Part II examination but who wish to use the Diploma examination as preparation for their membership examination. Candidates who have passed the MRCP(UK) Part I (Paediatrics) examination are exempted from the Diploma in Child Health Paper II (MCQ).

In contrast to MRCP(UK) Paeds Part II, the Diploma in Child Health examination neither tests detailed knowledge of in-patient care, nor knowledge of rare conditions. It tests knowledge, skill and competence of care (including basic principles of psychological and social aspects) of children in primary care.

Most candidates in the United Kingdom take the examination run by the Royal College of Physicians of London, and this revision book particularly helps candidates to revise for examination in this format.

The Royal Colleges in Glasgow and Dublin also run this Diploma examination. There are no multiple-choice question papers in these examinations.

There are two written papers held on the same day. The clinical examination takes place some weeks after the written examination, and only those who pass the multiple-choice questions paper are invited to attend the clinical examination.

Written section

Written paper I – 3 hours

10 short note questions – 50% (5% each)
Two case commentaries – 25% each

Written paper II – 2 hours

60 multiple-choice questions
Candidates must pass this paper before they are allowed to proceed to the clinical section.

Clinical section

Long case – 40 minutes with the patient and 20 minutes with the examiners
Short cases – Total 30 minutes
10 minutes – developmental assessment (including hearing or vision tests)
20 minutes – several short cases

GENERAL ADVICE ON TACKLING SHORT NOTE QUESTIONS

The examination format

The written paper will be marked only if you have obtained sufficient marks in the multiple-choice questions. You will automatically fail the whole examination if you have a clear fail in the multiple-choice question paper.

In the written paper, there are 10 short note questions and two case commentaries to be answered in 3 hours. It is recommended that you spend 90 minutes on the short note questions and 90 minutes on the two case commentaries.

Therefore, you will have 9 minutes for each short note question.

How to tackle the questions

The questions are usually of two types. The first type is a straightforward theoretical question asking for a list of causes, clinical features, investigations, management or prognosis. The second more common type asks how you would manage certain common clinical conditions.

The paper is scored according to the number of correct relevant points you identify. As time is limited, you should answer the questions in note form, preferably as a list. It is important to answer all the stems posed in each question. It is also important to adhere strictly to the available time of 9 minutes per question. You will have obtained most of the marks in the first few minutes, and spending a longer time on each question will not earn you many more marks, and you may run out of time on other questions. As a rough guide, 100 words is adequate for most questions.

We would suggest the following approach.

1 Identify all the stems to be answered

Example:

What are the characteristic features of toddler diarrhoea? What advice regarding management and prognosis would you give to the parents?

There are three stems to the questions.

A   A list of the characteristic features of toddler diarrhoea.
B   A list of advice to parents on the management.
C   A list of advice to parents on the prognosis.

2 Note the key words

In stem **A** in the above example, note the key word **characteristic**. You should give only those features which are typical of the disorder, not rarely associated features. Characteristic features include the age group of the children affected.

3 Use headings and lists

This will save you time in writing out your answers. You need not write full sentences.

4 Answer only the questions posed

You will only be awarded marks for relevant questions. In the example above, discussing the possible aetiology of toddler diarrhoea will not give you extra marks.

5 Stick to the 9-minute time limit

ADVICE ON ANSWERING CASE COMMENTARIES

The total time allowed for paper I is 3 hours. The recommended time for answering the short notes questions is approximately 90 minutes. The recommended time for answering *each* case commentary is 45 minutes. *Each* case commentary accounts for 25% of the whole paper.

The case commentaries are usually common situations you would meet as general practitioners. The question usually gives a brief outline of the case, and then asks you how you would assess the case further, the differential diagnosis and subsequent management. Alternatively, you may be asked questions as the case unfolds. In this case, it is important to answer the question without being influenced by the subsequent information available.

There are usually between four and five questions for each case commentary. If the question asks you to list the investigations or differential diagnosis, simply list them. If it asks you to discuss, you need to give views for and against the issue. If you have sufficient time, you should write full sentences in this section. However, if you run out of time, it is best to write in note form and put down the important points.

If you are asked to give a differential diagnosis (e.g. for primary amenorrhoea), either give the diagnoses in a logical order (e.g. hypothalamic causes, pituitary causes, ovarian causes etc.), or give the diagnoses in the order of likelihood.

If you are asked about the management of a child (e.g. anorexia), you should always consider three aspects:

- **Physical** (e.g. treatment of systemic illness causing anorexia, prevention of adverse physical effect of anorexia etc.);
- **Psychological** (e.g. family therapy, individual therapy, cognitive behavioural therapy);
- **Social** (e.g. influenced by social values, such as the pressure to be a ballet dancer).

You should also think about the contribution of different members of the multi-professional teams, if appropriate. Examples are physiotherapists, occupational therapists, dieticians, nurses, educational psychologists, school teachers and social workers etc.

If you are asked about the advice you would give to a patient, consider, if appropriate,

- **Health education** (e.g. parental smoking);
- **Prevention** (e.g. immunisation, screening, antenatal diagnosis etc.).

You should answer the questions set rather than a general question. For example, if you are asked the differential diagnoses in a case of delayed puberty, only give those diagnoses which are applicable to the details of the case given, and not a general list of causes of delayed puberty.

TEST 1
Short Note and Case Commentary Questions

Paper I

Time allowed: 3 hours.

There are two sections to Paper I: 10 short note questions and two case histories.

Short note questions

(Recommended time for answering approximately 90 minutes.)

The 10 short note questions carry 50% of the total marks. All the short note questions carry equal marks. The two case histories carry 50% of the total marks (25% each).

Write short notes on the following subjects. Conciseness will be beneficial. Lists are acceptable.

1 How would you assess a 3-month old baby whose head circumference lies below the 3rd centile?
2 A mother suspects that her 3-year old daughter has a squint. How would you assess the child? How would you advise the mother?
3 A 10-year old girl presents with secondary enuresis. Discuss the differential diagnoses. What questions you would ask her parents and how would you manage the child?
4 A routine urine culture in a 6-month old boy showed more than 100 000 *E. coli* per cubic mm. How would you manage the child?
5 Write short notes on the consent to treat children under 16 years of age.
6 Briefly discuss the importance of childhood road traffic accidents. List the measures which may reduce the incidence of childhood road traffic accidents.
7 List the clinical features of atopic eczema in a 4-year old child. What treatments are available?
8 A 7-year old boy with known grand mal epilepsy presents in the Accident and Emergency Department with status epilepticus. Discuss your strategy in his management.
9 You have diagnosed diabetic ketoacidosis in a 10-year old with known insulin-dependent diabetes. Outline your immediate management of the child.
10 Discuss the indications for circumcision (excluding cultural and traditional reasons). What complications may occur?

Case commentary 1

(Recommended time for answering approximately 45 minutes.)

Read the following case history carefully. Then answer ALL the questions below. Please start your answers on a separate page.

You are called to see John aged 18 months who has a 10-day history of cough. During the preceding 2 days, he has become pyrexial and listless. He had a previous chest infection 3 months ago which was treated by your partner. This had been slow to resolve and had required two courses of antibiotics. An intermittent cough had been present since then.

He has a younger sister aged 5 months. His parents are separated and he lives with his mother, who claims income support. His mother is a heavy smoker. There is no significant family history of note. John's developmental milestones have been normal.

On examination, he looks underweight and a recent clinic weight lies on the 3rd centile. He is listless and pyrexial with a respiratory rate of 60 per minute. He has intercostal and subcostal recession and crepitations are heard throughout both lung fields. His heart rate is 160/minute, no murmurs are present and his liver is not enlarged.

1 Discuss the differential diagnosis. What is the immediate management?

John was admitted to a paediatric ward. A chest X-ray showed patchy consolidation in both lung fields and he was treated with intravenous antibiotics. He was noted to have abdominal distension, greasy offensive stools and early finger clubbing.

2 What is the most likely underlying diagnosis? What investigations should be carried out to confirm the diagnosis?
3 The investigation confirmed your suspected diagnosis.
   (a) What points would you raise when discussing John's management and prognosis with his mother?
   (b) List the professionals who will help John in his long-term management.
   (c) What contribution can the general practitioner make to his management?

Case commentary 2

(Recommended time for answering approximately 45 minutes.)

Read the following case history carefully. Then answer ALL the questions below. Please start your answer on a separate page.

Susan, a 10-year old girl, has been referred to you, her family practitioner, because the school nurse is concerned about her obesity. She is 132 cm in height (about the 25th centile) but weighs 55 kg (much above the 97th centile). Her school nurse also informs you that she has been distressed by teasing and name calling at school.

Her records show that her birth weight was normal, and she has no significant past medical history. Her father is of average weight for his height, but her mother is also obese. Her parents were divorced a year ago, and Susan lives with her mother.

Susan denies eating excessively at meal times or taking snacks. She is keen to lose weight. Her mother also tells you that she refused to attend school during the previous week. Physical examination confirms the height and weight measurements but she otherwise appears healthy.

1 Discuss the differential diagnosis of her obesity. What other information would you try to obtain, and what other physical signs would you look for?

2 What investigations would you arrange and why?

3 Assuming that all your investigations are normal, what advice and support would you give to Susan and her mother regarding her long-term management?

4 What factors might contribute to the problem of school refusal? How would you manage this problem?

TEST 2
Short Note and Case Commentary Questions

Paper I

Time allowed: 3 hours

There are 2 sections to Paper I: 10 short note questions and two case histories.

The 10 short note questions carry 50% of the total marks. All the short note questions carry equal marks. The 2 case histories carry 50% of the total marks (25% each).

Short note questions

(Recommended time for answering approximately 90 minutes.)

Write short notes on the following subjects. Conciseness will be beneficial. Lists are acceptable.

1 What are the risk factors for congenital dislocation of the hips? Briefly describe how you would screen for congenital dislocation of the hips in the neonatal period.

2 What are the criteria for a good screening test? Briefly describe the common screening test for two disorders which fulfil most of these criteria.

3 A 3-year old boy with known asthma presents in the Accident and Emergency Department with an acute asthmatic attack. List the signs and symptoms which would indicate the severity of this attack. What is your strategy for treating him?

4 A 16-year old girl presents with short stature and primary amenorrhoea. List the main causes and summarise your management of this girl.

5 You have a 5-year old patient with mild cerebral diplegia. What problems might he experience? List the professionals who may be involved in his care, and briefly list their roles.

6 A 9-year old boy presents with a 3-day history of fleeting joint pain, petechial rash over the buttocks, and abdominal pain. What is the most likely diagnosis? What are the other features and complications of this disorder?

7 A 4-year old boy is brought to you with speech delay. What are the possible causes, and how would you assess him?

8 List the clinical features of tuberous sclerosis in a child. What investigations would support your diagnosis?

9 What are the clinical signs of a ventricular septal defect? How would you evaluate the size of the defect clinically in a 3-month old child? How would you manage the child?

10 What are the features of bruising associated with non-accidental injury? What conditions might be confused with non-accidental bruising?

Case commentary 1

(Recommended time for answering approximately 45 minutes.)

Read the following case history carefully. Then answer ALL the questions below. Please start your answers on a separate page.

Fred, a 2-year old boy, is brought by his mother to see you because of his temper tantrums. His mother says that whenever he does not have his way, he will shout, scream and throw toys until his demands are met. On two occasions during the previous week, he stopped breathing and became blue and unconscious shortly after temper tantrums. He recovered rapidly and spontaneously, but his parents are very worried that he may have epilepsy.

Fred was born at 37 weeks gestation with a birth weight of 3.2 kg. His records show that his developmental milestones were normal. His father is a teacher, and his mother a part-time secretary. Both are Caucasian. Fred is the only child in the family. There is no significant family history of note.

On physical examination, he looks pale, but there are no other abnormal findings and he is thriving.

1 What is the likely diagnosis for the two recent episodes described by his mother? What advice would you give regarding the investigation, treatment and prognosis of these episodes?

2 Discuss a management strategy for his temper tantrum.

You arrange for his haemoglobin to be checked. The result comes back as 8 g/dl.

3 Discuss the most likely cause of his anaemia. How would you investigate further?

4 Discuss your management of the most likely cause of his anaemia.

Case commentary 2

(Recommended time for answering approximately 45 minutes.)

Read the following case history carefully. Then answer ALL the questions below. Please start your answers on a separate page.

Jack, an 8-month old boy, is brought to see you because of episodes during which his head and trunk are suddenly thrown forwards. These are associated with flexion of his arms and legs and occur in clusters of between 10 to 20 episodes. Each episode lasts a few seconds only. They had their onset about 2 weeks previously.

Jack was born at term by normal delivery weighing 3.5 kg. Apgar scores were 8 at 1 minute and 9 at 5 minutes. His developmental checks at 6 weeks, 3 months and 6 months were satisfactory. There is no significant family history of note. He is the only child, but his parents are planning to have more children. Both parents are managers at a large manufacturing company.

On examination, he is quiet and subdued. Jack is afebrile. His anterior fontanelle is normotensive. There are no skin lesions. Neurological examination is unremarkable, and his development is compatible with his chronological age.

1   What is the diagnosis?
2   What investigation would you perform to confirm your diagnosis? What would you expect to find?
3   What are the possible underlying causes for this condition?
4   What other investigations should be performed to look for underlying causes?
5   Briefly describe Jack's management.
6   What is his prognosis?
7   What advice would you give his parents regarding future children?

TEST 3
Short Note and Case Commentary Questions

Paper I

Time allowed: 3 hours

There are two sections to Paper I: 10 short note questions and two case histories. The 10 short note questions carry 50% of the total marks. All the short note questions carry equal marks. The two case histories carry 50% of the total marks (25% each).

Short note questions

(Recommended time for answering approximately 90 minutes.)

Write short notes on the following subjects. Conciseness will be beneficial. Lists are acceptable.

1 What are the advantages of administering the MMR (measles, mumps and rubella) immunisation to the health of the population and the child receiving the vaccine? What are the possible side-effects ?

2 You are asked to see a 12-hour old neonate with clinical jaundice. What are the likely causes and how would you investigate and manage the child?

3 List the possible causes of faecal soiling. How would you manage a 5-year old boy with recent onset of faecal soiling?

4 A 4-year old boy presents with recent onset of bruises. What is the differential diagnosis and how would you investigate the child?

5 A 12-month old boy presents with a 2-week history of persistent pyrexia, cervical lymphadenopathy, mouth ulceration, and recent peeling of the palms. What is the most likely diagnosis? List the clinical features and possible complications and briefly describe how he should be managed.

6 List the characteristic features of acute bacterial meningitis in a 9-month old boy. List the common organisms responsible and possible complications.

7 A 3-year old boy presents with a first episode of typical febrile convulsion lasting 2 minutes. How would you assess and manage the child? What advice would you give to his parents?

8 You were unable to palpate the testes of a male newborn infant during routine examination. What are the possible causes and how would you manage the child?

9 What are the characteristic features of toddler diarrhoea? What advice regarding management and prognosis would you give to the parents?

10 What problems are encountered by children born with cleft lip and palate? What is the paediatrician's role in the management of the condition?

Case commentary 1

(Recommended time for answering approximately 45 minutes.)

Read the following case history carefully. Then answer ALL the questions below. Please start your answers on a separate page.

Sarah, a 12-year old girl, is brought to see you, her family practitioner, by her parents who are concerned about her short stature. She has always been the shortest in the class, but the difference in height between Sarah and her peers has become more noticeable recently.

Your records show that her height and weight were on the 3rd centile lines at 5 years of age. Sarah weighed 2.9 kg at birth, and had an uneventful neonatal period. She has no significant past medical or family history. She has two older brothers both of whom are said to be of average height. She is usually a happy and lively girl, but has recently become increasingly unhappy about her short stature.

Examination reveals a short pleasant cooperative girl. Her height of 126 cm and her weight of 27 kg both lie below the 3rd centile lines. She is pre-pubertal, with no signs of breast, axillary hair or pubic hair development.

1 Discuss the differential diagnosis of Sarah's short stature.

2 What further information would you seek? What would you look for on physical examination and what investigations would you consider?

You decided to refer Sarah to the local paediatrician. Eight weeks later, Sarah and her parents consulted you again in a distressed state. They told you that after blood tests and X-rays, they were seen by the paediatrician yesterday who told them that Sarah had a disorder called 'Turner's syndrome', and that she would require hormonal treatment. However, they did not fully understand what the paediatrician was telling them. You had just received a brief letter from the paediatrician the same day confirming this diagnosis, and indicating that he planned to treat Sarah with growth hormone in addition to oestrogen.

3 How would you explain this condition and the proposed treatment to Sarah and her parents?

4 Are there any other issues which you would wish to raise with Sarah and her parents?

Case commentary 2

(Recommended time for answering approximately 45 minutes.)

Read the following case history carefully. Then answer ALL the questions below. Please start your answers on a separate page.

A couple brought their 3-year old son Tom to see you, his family general practitioner, and asked you to prescribe a hypnotic for him. In the last year, Tom has refused to go to bed at the appropriate time. He would stay up late and insist on going to his parents' bed rather than his own. If put to bed, he would scream and shout until his parents took him downstairs again 5 minutes later. He would often wake up in the middle of the night demanding his parents' attention.

Tom had a normal birth, and there was no significant family or past medical history. He has a younger sister aged 13 months. His father is a taxi driver and works irregular hours. His mother is a part-time cleaner in the evening, and both parents find Tom's behaviour tiring and unbearable. They are also worried that Tom's lack of sleep may be due to an underlying serious illness.

Physical examination reveals a healthy 4-year old child with normal developmental milestones and no abnormal physical findings apart from dental caries.

1 What factors may have contributed to Tom's sleeping problems?
2 What advice and treatment would you give Tom's parents regarding his sleep problems?
3 What advice would you give his parents regarding his dental caries?

TEST 4
Short Note and Case Commentary Questions

Paper I

Time allowed: 3 hours

There are two sections to Paper I: 10 short note questions and two case histories.

The 10 short note questions carry 50% of the total marks. All the short note questions carry equal marks. The two case histories carry 50% of the total marks (25% each).

Short note questions

(Recommended time for answering approximately 90 minutes.)

Write short notes on the following subjects. Conciseness will be beneficial. Lists are acceptable.

1 Describe how you would assess failure to thrive in a 2-year old child with known asthma whose weight is below the 3rd centile.
2 What are the causes of precocious puberty? How would you assess a 7-year old girl with the onset of puberty?
3 List the advantages and disadvantages of breast-feeding compared with bottle feeding.
4 A 10-year 6-month old girl with a good academic record presents with 3 weeks' history of refusing to go to school. What are the possible causes? How would you manage the child?
5 Write short notes on the following:
   (a) Strawberry naevus
   (b) Café-au-lait spots
6 What basic principles underpin the changes contained in the 1989 Children Act?
7 You are called to see a 9-month old child with gastroenteritis. What are the clinical features of dehydration? What questions would you ask the parents? Briefly describe how you would manage the child.
8 What are the common organisms causing chest infection in a 5-year old boy for the first time? How would you treat him?

9 Severe haemophilia A has been diagnosed in a 1-month old boy whose grandfather, a haemophiliac, died from an intracranial haemorrhage 26 years ago. He is the first child of the couple. What points would you raise in discussions with his parents?

10 What is the definition of juvenile chronic arthritis? How would you classify the disorder?

Case commentary 1

(Recommended time for answering approximately 45 minutes.)

Read the following case history carefully. Then answer ALL the questions below. Please start your answers on a separate page.

You are asked to visit Jack, a 5-year old boy, at home urgently at 8:30 pm by his parents. According to his mother, he appeared to be well and was playing on his own in the afternoon while his father was out at work and she was cleaning in the house. However, in the early evening, he had become increasingly drowsy, and could not be aroused by 8 pm. His parents were particularly concerned because a child at Jack's school had been admitted to hospital 5 days ago with a presumptive diagnosis of meningitis.

Jack had no significant past medical history. His perinatal history had been uneventful and his developmental milestones normal. His immunisation status was up to date. His father suffered from a severe generalised anxiety disorder, but his mother had no significant medical problems.

On examination, Jack was unarousable. His temperature was 37 °C. He had diminished tone in all his limbs with absent reflexes. He did not have neck stiffness.

1 What other points in the history would you elicit and what physical signs would you look for?
2 List the differential diagnoses.
3 What would be your immediate management as a general practitioner?

Jack was admitted to hospital. When you visited him in hospital at 8 am the next morning, you were told that so far investigations (which included a CT scan) were normal, and that Jack had regained consciousness. You found him playing happily with other children.

4 What was the most likely diagnosis?
5 What advice should be given to his parents when he is discharged from hospital?

Case commentary 2

(Recommended time for answering approximately 45 minutes.)

Read the following case history carefully. Then answer ALL the questions below. Please start your answer on a separate page.

Sarah, a 10-month old, was admitted after being brought to the Accident and Emergency Department with a history of two episodes of passing bright red blood in her urine. She was a first child, born at term, weighing 3.8 kg. The perinatal period and development had been uneventful and she had no previous illnesses of note. Her mother was a 25-year old, unmarried, former care assistant in an old people's home. She was noted to be quiet and inhibited. Her father was 26 years old and unemployed. He was aggressive and demanded immediate answers. Physical examination including BP, genitalia and anus was normal.

1   Discuss your assessment and investigation of this case.

Investigations proved to be normal and the baby remained well. Repeated urinalyses were normal. On several occasions, her mother, who remained anxious, produced nappies containing fresh blood, although the nursing staff reported no blood when the parents were absent. Her father remained aggressive and hostile. On one occasion, her parents complained about lack of privacy and demanded a change of room.

2   What is the likely diagnosis?
3   What steps should be taken at this point?
4   What further information might be helpful?
5   What points would you raise at a subsequent case conference? How can this family be helped?

TEST 5
Short Note and Case Commentary Questions

Paper I

Time allowed: 3 hours

There are two sections to Paper I: 10 short note questions and two case histories.

The 10 short note questions carry 50% of the total marks. All the short note questions carry equal marks. The two case histories carry 50% of the total marks (25% each).

Short note questions

(Recommended time for answering approximately 90 minutes.)

Write short notes on the following subjects. Conciseness will be beneficial. Lists are acceptable.

1 A systolic murmur was noted on routine examination of a 2-year old boy who otherwise appears healthy. List the clinical features which would suggest underlying congenital cardiac abnormality and the clinical features which would suggest that this is an innocent murmur.

2 What are the risk factors for deafness in a child? Describe the routine screening test in infancy for deafness, and state when the test should be performed.

3 List the clinical signs of Down's syndrome. What other conditions may be associated with Down's syndrome?

4 What are the characteristic clinical features of nephrotic syndrome? What investigations would confirm this diagnosis and elucidate the underlying cause for the nephrotic syndrome?

5 A 6-week old male infant presents with projectile vomiting after every feed, but appears hungry afterwards. What is the most likely diagnosis? List the possible biochemical abnormalities. How would you confirm the diagnosis? What is the treatment?

6 A healthy 8-year old boy was found to have a random blood pressure measurement of 140/110. What are the possible causes? What investigations would you perform?

7 A 7-year old child presents with a bald patch on his scalp. What are the possible causes? Briefly describe the treatment for each cause.

8 Discuss the presentation, management and diagnosis of intussusception.

9 What clinical features would make you suspect Duchenne muscular dystrophy in a 4-year old boy? What is his likely prognosis? What points are important in discussing management with his parents?

10 List the problems which may be encountered during the first year of life by a baby born to an HIV positive mother. What advice would you give regarding immunisation?

Case commentary 1

(Recommended time for answering approximately 45 minutes.)

Read the following case history carefully. Then answer ALL the questions below. Please start your answers on a separate page.

Matthew, aged 4 weeks, is brought to see you by his parents in your surgery. Although he has fed well, Matthew has been vomiting after feeds since the end of his first week after birth.

   Matthew is their second child. He was born at term and had an uneventful perinatal period. His weight and head circumference have continued to lie on the 50th centile lines since birth. He has been bottle-fed since birth.

1 What is the most likely diagnosis? What other diagnoses would you consider? Describe how you would assess the situation.

You reassure the parents and decide to thicken his feeds with Carobel. Three weeks later, you are asked to see Matthew again because of a choking episode unrelated to feeding. His parents also tell you that he has had a cough and sounded 'rattly' for 2 weeks.

2 What investigations should be carried out at this point?
3 Outline your management strategy.

Case commentary 2

(Recommended time for answering approximately 45 minutes.)

Read the following case history carefully. Then answer ALL the questions below. Please start your answers on a separate page.

Louise, a 12-year old girl, has been brought to see you because of frequent episodes of central abdominal pain and poor appetite. She had been well with no previous illness of note until 3 months ago. She has not lost any time from school because of her symptoms. Her mother says she is of average academic ability, but is a quiet and conscientious child.

   Her father died 18 months ago of lymphoma, and she lives alone with her mother, a full-time legal secretary. Her 19-year old brother is away from home at university.

   On examination, she is pre-pubertal, but looks well with no abnormal findings. Her height of 134 cm is just below the 3rd centile, while her weight of 30 kg is on the 3rd centile. Her mother is 152.5 cm while her father was 165 cm.

1   What specific questions would you ask regarding her abdominal pain?

2   What further information would you try to obtain?

3   What investigations would you carry out at this stage and why?

All investigations prove to be normal. When she is seen again 6 weeks later, she still complains of abdominal pain. Examination is again normal, and she has gained weight.

4   Discuss your future management of this case.

ADVICE ON ANSWERING MULTIPLE-CHOICE QUESTIONS

Written Paper II is a 60 multiple-choice question paper lasting 2 hours. If you do not pass this paper, Paper I will not be marked, and you are not allowed to proceed to the clinical examination.

Each question has a stem followed by five items marked **A** to **E**. You are required to answer whether each of the items **A** to **E** is true or false. You can also respond by filling in the 'don't know' box. You score plus 1 mark for a correct answer, −1 mark for an incorrect answer, and 0 mark for 'don't know'. As the pass score varies from one examination to another, you should aim for as high a score as possible.

It is debatable what the best strategy is if you do not know the answer. Statistically, a total random guess to some questions should not affect your score, and you should on the whole improve your score if you attempt the questions you are not sure of by an educated guess. However, it may be true that some are better than others at guessing.

In the examination, try to answer the questions reasonably quickly, marking those you are not sure of. You can then return to these afterwards. Allow plenty of time to transfer your answers to the answer sheet provided.

TEST 1
Multiple-Choice Questions

Time allowed: 2 hours
  Each question consists of an initial statement (stem) followed by five completions (items) marked A to E. Each item may be true or false, and in the examination, it is possible for the five items in any question to be all true or all false, or any intermediate combination.
  One mark (+ 1) will be awarded for each correct answer. One mark will be deducted (– 1) for each incorrect answer. A zero (0) mark will be awarded for each 'don't know' (DK) answer.

1 The Court Report

  A was published in 1946.
  B recommended a multi-professional team in each health district for the treatment of handicapped children.
  C recommended that there is at least one community consultant paediatrician with special skills in developmental, social and educational paediatrics in each health district.
  D recommended that the child health visitor should be involved with preventative but not curative aspects of child health.
  E has been fully implemented.

2 Which of the following statements describe the philosophy of education of children with special educational needs in the 1990s?

  A The type of education required depends on the cause of the disability.
  B The type of education required depends on the child's intelligence quotient.
  C The curriculum provided should be different from that provided to other children.
  D The education provided should be focused on the child's disability.
  E Only teachers with special educational needs teaching qualifications should teach the child.

3 The provision of sex education

  A must take place in all schools.
  B is decided by the headteachers in consultation with all teachers in schools.
  C should take into account cultural differences.
  D must be undertaken by science teachers.
  E should be different in content for children with special needs.

4 Factors associated with successful foster placements include
  A children of older age group.
  B a short period of being in care.
  C the presence of children of a similar age group in the placement family.
  D the child's enthusiasm to be placed in foster care.
  E separation from familiar background.

5 Which of the following definitions are correct?
  A Stillbirth rate is the number of babies born dead with a gestational age of at least 24 weeks (previously 28 weeks) per 1000 live births.
  B Perinatal mortality rate is the number of babies who die in the first 7 days of life per 1000 live births.
  C Infant mortality rate is the number of infants dying in the first 12 months of life per 1000 total births.
  D Neonatal mortality rate is the number of babies dying in the first 28 days of life per 1000 live births.
  E Post-neonatal mortality rate is the number of babies who die between 28 days and 1 year per 1000 live births.

6 The following statements are true regarding child health clinics.
  A They are staffed mainly by community paediatricians.
  B Immunisations are given in child health clinics.
  C Health education is carried out in child health clinics.
  D Developmental assessments are carried out.
  E They render home visiting unnecessary.

7 Parent-held records in relation to child health surveillance
  A are often lost by parents.
  B enhance communication between health professionals and parents.
  C encourage parents to become involved.
  D are generally preferred by parents compared with clinic-held records.
  E are generally not favoured by general practitioners compared with clinic-held records.

8 Oral polio vaccine
  A is contraindicated in pregnancy.
  B is contraindicated in those with immunodeficiency.
  C may rarely result in polio in vaccine contacts.
  D consists of a mixture of three live attenuated strains of virus.
  E is excreted in faeces.

9 Pertussis vaccine

A is a killed vaccine.
B should not be given to any children who have developed pyrexia following a previous dose.
C should not be given to any children who developed a severe reaction to a preceding dose.
D is contraindicated in cystic fibrosis.
E is usually combined with tetanus and diphtheria vaccines.

10 Which of the following foods are appropriate for the child?

A Skimmed milk for a 12-month old child.
B Chocolate cakes as snacks for a 3-year old child.
C Fresh fruits as snacks for a 4-year old child.
D Highly salted fish for a 2-year old.
E Wholemeal bread for a 4-year old.

11 Growth hormone deficiency

A may present with hyperglycaemia.
B may cause genital abnormalities in the affected neonate.
C may be associated with other endocrine deficiencies.
D may be associated with obesity.
E may be treated with subcutaneous human growth hormone replacement.

12 The average 9-month old baby is able to

A sit unsupported for 2 minutes.
B walk around the furniture.
C roll from supine to prone position.
D transfer an object from one hand to another.
E approach objects with the index finger.

13 Physical signs strongly suggestive of child physical abuse include

A forehead bruising in a toddler.
B torn frenulum.
C generalised purpuric rash.
D retinal haemorrhages.
E multiple bruises of differing ages on the shins of an 8-year old boy.

14 Tympanometry

A is a reliable test for hearing.
B detects sensori-neural deafness.
C measures middle ear pressure.
D can be performed on a 3-year old child.
E is regarded as normal if the curve is flat.

15 The following observations support a diagnosis of non-accidental injury.

   A The parents appear overprotective of the child.
   B Unexplained delay in seeking medical advice.
   C Generalised bruises.
   D Torn frenulum.
   E Fracture of tibia in a 9-month old baby.

16 The following features are characteristic of Kawasaki's disease (mucocutaneous lymph node syndrome).

   A Peeling of the palms.
   B Prolonged pyrexia.
   C Low platelets.
   D Cervical lymphanopathy
   E Purulent conjunctival discharge.

17 The following statements are true regarding interpretation of the Mantoux test.

   A A negative response excludes active tuberculosis.
   B A wheal of more than 1.5 cm suggests active tuberculosis.
   C A wheal of 4 mm indicates a positive test.
   D A wheal of 1 cm may be due to previous BCG immunisation.
   E It is less reliable than the Heaf test.

18 The following problems are more common in babies who are small for their gestational age.

   A Hypoglycaemia.
   B Hypothermia.
   C Anaemia
   D Congenital abnormality.
   E Respiratory distress syndrome.

19 The following are causes of unconjugated hyperbilirubinaemia.

   A Physiological jaundice.
   B Rhesus disease.
   C Neonatal hepatitis.
   D Biliary atresia.
   E Breast-milk jaundice.

✱ 20 The following are examples of secondary prevention.

   A Immunisation for whooping cough.
   B Neonatal screening for hypothyroidism.
   C Preconceptual genetic counselling.
   D Addition of fluoride to drinking water.
   E Amniocentesis to diagnose Down's syndrome.

21 An average 2-year old child can

A go upstairs two feet per step.
B go downstairs one foot per step.
C give his or her full name
D build a tower of six cubes.
E copy a circle with pencil.

22 The following statements about coeliac disease are true.

A It predominantly affects the distal small intestine.
B There is an increased incidence in those with a family history of the disease.
C It usually presents before 7 months of age.
D It may cause anaemia.
E Jejunal biopsy may help in its diagnosis.

23 The following statements on chronic constipation in childhood are true.

A It is more likely to be caused by congenital abnormality of the bowel the younger the child presents.
B Most children with chronic constipation have no organic pathology.
C A stimulant laxative and stool softener may be used together.
D Simple behavioural programmes may be effective.
E Dietary factors are important.

24 The following infections are causes of pneumonia in the immuno-compromised child.

A Chickenpox.
B Measles.
C *Pneumocystis.*
D Herpes simplex.
E Cytomegalovirus.

25 The following statements about the use of sodium cromoglycate in asthma are true.

A It can be given orally.
B It can be used as a first-line prophylactic drug.
C It can inhibit growth.
D It may be given four times daily.
E It can be used to treat an acute attack.

26 The following statements about asthma in children are correct.

A Inhaled salbutamol immediately before exercise is effective in preventing exercise-induced attack.
B Sodium cromoglycate may be useful in preventing seasonal asthma.
C Inhaled steroid may be useful in preventing seasonal asthma.
D Symptoms at night may indicate that the disease is poorly controlled.
E Peak flow measurement is an effective method of monitoring the disease for children aged 7 and older.

27 Acute epiglottitis

   A is most often caused by *Haemophilus influenzae* Type B.
   B commonly occurs in infants below 1 year of age.
   C should be diagnosed by inspection of the throat.
   D is characteristically associated with drooling of saliva.
   E should be diagnosed by a lateral neck X-ray.

28 The following are important signs to look for in the assessment of heart disease in infants.

   A Enlarged liver.
   B Raised jugular venous pressure.
   C Ankle oedema.
   D Tachycardia.
   E Presence of femoral pulses.

29 The following findings are compatible with an innocent murmur.

   A Fixed splitting of the second heart sound.
   B The murmur varies with the position of the child.
   C A diastolic murmur.
   D A Grade 4/6 murmur.
   E A high-pitched murmur.

30 Risk factors for congenital heart disease include

   A Down's syndrome.
   B Turner's syndrome.
   C a family history of congenital heart disease.
   E maternal diabetes.
   E maternal alcohol consumption.

31 Causes of secondary hypertension include

   A chronic glomerulonephritis.
   B coarctation of the aorta.
   C Wilms' tumour.
   D phaeochromocytoma.
   E pulmonary stenosis.

32 Recurrent febrile convulsions

   A are more likely to be prolonged than the first convulsion.
   B are more likely to occur if the first convulsion was prolonged.
   C occur in about one-third of children with a previous febrile convulsion.
   D can be prevented by giving phenobarbitone during febrile illnesses.
   E should always be prevented following two or more febrile convulsions by giving long-term anticonvulsants.

33 Migraine

   A occurs in less than 1% of school children.
   B is more common in boys than in girls before the age of 11.
   C becomes more common with age in girls.
   D is more common in children with a positive family history.
   E may be triggered by exercise in some children.

34 Hemiplegic cerebral palsy

   A may be the result of an intrauterine thromboembolic event.
   B is rarely associated with seizures.
   C is associated with mental retardation in most cases.
   D often affects the leg more than the arm.
   E may cause shortening of the affected leg.

35 Tuberous sclerosis

   A is autosomal recessive in inheritance.
   B may be diagnosed by a CT scan of the brain.
   C may present with epilepsy.
   D can be asymptomatic.
   E is frequently associated with adenoma sebaceum (facial angiofibromata) in infancy.

36 Haemophilia A

   A has an autosomal recessive inheritance.
   B is usually associated with a prolonged prothrombin time.
   C may be diagnosed antenatally in those with a previously affected child.
   D should be treated with aspirin for pain due to haemarthrosis.
   E may be treated prophylactically with desmopressin (DDAVP) in mild cases before minor surgical procedures.

37 Recognised features of acute glomerulonephritis include

   A oedema.
   B hypertension.
   C haematuria.
   D polyuria.
   E frequency.

38 Growth hormone deficiency

   A is an all-or-nothing phenomenon.
   B may be acquired.
   C can be diagnosed by a random growth hormone level.
   D may temporarily result from psychosocial deprivation.
   E is treated by twice weekly subcutaneous injections of growth hormone.

39 Children with diabetic ketoacidosis

    A may present with abdominal pain.
    B should be fluid restricted.
    C should be given long-acting insulin immediately.
    D may develop cerebral oedema.
    E should be given dextrose 4%, saline 0.18% initially.

40 Signs associated with a severe degree of dehydration include

    A high fever.
    B bulging fontanelle in infants.
    C normal skin turgor.
    D failure to pass urine.
    E metabolic acidosis.

41 Scabies

    A is caused by mites.
    B treatment should be offered only to family members who have symptoms.
    C commonly causes intense nocturnal itching.
    D is frequently transmitted via clothing.
    E may be complicated by impetigo.

42 The following findings are consistent with an innocent murmur.

    A A soft murmur in the pulmonary area.
    B A vibratory ejection systolic murmur heard at the left lower sternal edge.
    C A pansystolic murmur heard at the left lower sternal edge.
    D Fixed splitting of the second heart sound.
    E A continuous murmur heard below the clavicle which varies with the position of the head.

43 The following biochemical findings are characteristic of congenital hypertrophic pyloric stenosis.

    A Low chloride.
    B Low bicarbonate.
    C Low pH.
    D High potassium.
    E High glucose.

44 Coeliac disease in children

    A may present with short stature and no gastrointestinal symptoms.
    B can now be diagnosed by measuring circulating IgA gliadin, IgA antireticulin and IgA anti-endomysial antibodies.
    C is associated with an increased risk of lymphoma if untreated.
    D is associated with IgA deficiency.
    E should be treated by excluding wheat, rye, barley and oats from the diet.

45 The incidence of vertical transmission of HIV infection from mother to baby

A is more than 75% in Europe.
B is decreased if the mother takes AZT in pregnancy.
C is increased in babies born before 34 weeks gestation.
D is increased in mothers with symptomatic HIV infection.
E is increased in mothers with low T4 cell counts.

46 In children with HIV infection

A lymphoid interstitial pneumonitis is associated with a bad prognosis.
B bacterial infections occur more frequently than in HIV infected adults.
C infection with *Pneumocystic carnii* carries a poor prognosis.
D Kaposi sarcoma occurs at some stage in 30% of infected children.
E all immunisations are contraindicated.

47 Intussusception

A occurs mainly in children over 5 years of age.
B occurs more often in boys than girls.
C is ileo-colic in most cases.
D may present with symptoms suggesting neurological disease.
E may be diagnosed by abdominal ultrasonography.

48 In children, a prolonged bleeding time occurs in

A haemophilia A.
B Von Willebrand's disease.
C aspirin ingestion.
D Christmas disease.
E idiopathic thrombocytopenic purpura.

49 Precocious puberty

A is more common in boys.
B is likely to be associated with intracranial tumours in girls.
C causes an increase in the final height.
D is commonly associated with a delayed bone age.
E is associated with an enlarged uterus in girls.

50 There is a recognised association between

A Wilms tumour and aniridia.
B asthma and gastro-oesophageal reflux.
C Tuberous sclerosis and café au lait macules.
D subacute sclerosing panencephalitis and early infection with measles.
E Wilms tumour and hemihypertrophy.

51 Congenital hypertrophic pyloric stenosis

  A is present at birth.
  B is more common in girls.
  C causes bile stained vomiting.
  D is a recognised cause of haematemesis.
  E may be complicated by gastro-oesophageal reflux.

52 Infantile spasms

  A most often have their onset between 8 and 15 months.
  B may be an early manifestation of tuberous sclerosis.
  C are associated with mental retardation in 40% of cases.
  D may respond to vigabatrin.
  E should be treated with corticosteroids because these drugs improve the long term outcome.

53 The following may occur in infants of diabetic mothers.

  A Polycythaemia.
  B Ventricular septal defect.
  C Hypercalcaemia.
  D An increased incidence of respiratory distress syndrome.
  E An increased incidence of renal vein thrombosis.

54 Boys with X-linked hypogammaglobulinaemia

  A usually become symptomatic between 2 and 3 years of age.
  B usually have splenomegaly.
  C may develop bronchiectasis.
  D may develop echovirus encephalitis.
  E should be referred for bone marrow transplant.

55 Duchenne muscular dystrophy

  A is inherited as an autosomal recessive condition.
  B may present with mental handicap.
  C often causes delay in walking.
  D is associated with elevated creatinine kinase at birth.
  E causes a loss in the ability to walk between 15 and 20 years of age.

56 In juvenile chronic arthritis

  A joint pain and swelling should be present for 6 weeks before the diagnosis is made.
  B the most common onset is an illness with fever, rash and lymphadenopathy.
  C tests for rheumatoid factor are helpful in making the diagnosis.
  D the presence of anti-nuclear antibodies indicate a significant risk of chronic uveitis.
  E most children will have chronic joint disease in adult life.

57 In cow's milk protein intolerance

   A a negative skin test to cows' milk makes the diagnosis unlikely.
   B wheezing as the sole symptom occurs rarely.
   C the condition may follow gastroenteritis.
   D gastrointestinal symptoms are the most common.
   E a small intestinal biopsy may show partial villous atrophy.

58 Congenital hypothyroidism

   A affects approximately 1 in 4000 infants.
   B is most often due to an inborn error of thyroxine synthesis.
   C may be a transient phenomenon.
   D is more common in babies with Down's syndrome.
   E is associated with an IQ in the normal range in patients diagnosed within the first 6 weeks of life.

59 Osteomyelitis in children

   A is most commonly acquired by the haematogenous route.
   B may be caused by *Haemophilus influenzae*.
   C most commonly affects the lower tibia.
   D causes radiological abnormalities during the first 5 days of illness.
   E should be treated with antibiotics for 2 weeks.

60 Physiological jaundice

   A occurs in 5 to 10% of normal term babies.
   B is often apparent in the first 24 to 48 hours of life.
   C may be present for 2 to 3 weeks.
   D may cause vomiting.
   E may cause dark urine and pale stools.

TEST 2
Multiple-Choice Questions

Time allowed: 2 hours
 Each question consists of an initial statement (stem) followed by five completions (items) marked A to E. Each item may be true or false, and in the examination, it is possible for the five items in any question to be all true or all false, or any intermediate combination.
 One mark (+1) will be awarded for each correct answer. One mark will be deducted (−1) for each incorrect answer. A zero mark will be awarded for each 'don't know' (DK) answer.

1 The Child Development Centre

 A must be provided in the community and not on the hospital site.
 B assesses children with learning difficulties.
 C assesses children with physical disabilities.
 D should provide accommodation for occupation therapists, speech thera-
    pists, and psychologists.
 E should provide accommodation for a peripatetic service.

2 Which of the following statements describe the philosophy of education of
  children with special educational needs in the 1990s?

 A The child should be placed in a school appropriate to his or her diagnostic
    label.
 B Children with the same diagnostic label may have different educational
    needs.
 C All children in the same class should be taught at the same rate.
 D All children in the same class should be taught by the same method.
 E Streaming of students in a class is essential.

3 The following statements regarding day-care facilities for children are
  true.

 A A significant proportion of the day nurseries are run by social services
    departments.
 B Day nurseries are staffed by nursery nurses who must undergo a 2-year
    training course.
 C Family centres aim to increase the confidence of parents.
 D Family centres aim to teach parents parenting skills.
 E Playgroups need not be registered with the local authorities.

4 The following statements about adoption are true.

A The number of adoptions has increased in the last decade.
B The rights of the adopting parents are of paramount importance.
C Adoption can be arranged by any individuals.
D Adopted children have the right of access to their original birth certificates after the age of 18.
E Step-parents may apply to adopt the child.

5 The following are examples of secondary prevention.

A Screening for congenital dislocation of the hips.
B Screening for galactosaemia.
C Stabilising brittle diabetes.
D Enforcing the law regarding seat-belts for children.
E Immunisation against tetanus.

6 The following are essential components of an effective school health surveillance system.

A Regular routine physical examinations by the school doctors for all students.
B Routine physical examination by the school doctors for all students at entrance.
C A dedicated clinic outside the school.
D A named school nurse and doctor for every school.
E A good working relationship between teachers and school health team.

7 The following infectious diseases are notifiable in the United Kingdom.

A Mumps.
B Rubella.
C Streptococcal infection.
D Whooping cough.
E Scabies.

8 Measles

A is a notifiable disease in the United Kingdom.
B causes a maculopapular rash which appears initially behind the ears.
C is associated with Koplik's spots which characteristically appear after the onset of rash.
D may cause encephalitis.
E is associated with subacute sclerosing panencephalitis.

9 *Haemophilus influenzae* Type B

A is the main cause of epiglottitis.
B is the main cause of croup.
C is an encapsulated organism.
D causes meningitis with a high rate of neurological sequele.
E may complicate chest infection in cystic fibrosis.

10 Toddler diarrhoea

   A may occur at 18 months of age.
   B is often accompanied by failure to thrive.
   C is the passage of frequent loose stools with undigested food particles.
   D may occur in children who drink excessive amounts of juices.
   E may be treated with loperamide.

11 Growth retardation due to psychological deprivation

   A can be diagnosed with a biochemical test.
   B is excluded by a reduced growth hormone response to a stimulation test.
   C may reverse when the child is placed in a different environment.
   D is more common than isolated growth hormone deficiency.
   E can be easily managed.

12 The average 18-month old child can

   A kick a ball.
   B build a tower of two cubes.
   C show anxiety towards strangers.
   D imitate drawing a circle.
   E wave bye-bye.

13 The following are true about the visual screening of children.

   A If visual acuity is normal at school entry, re-testing at later ages is un-
     necessary.
   B A newborn baby can follow a dangling object horizontally for 180°.
   C Single letters are preferable to linear Snellen chart for a 3-year old
     child.
   D Children born very prematurely require special attention.
   E Squints can be excluded in a 3-month old baby by a cover test performed
     by the general practitioner.

14 The clumsy child syndrome (developmental dyspraxia)

   A is associated with left-handedness.
   B may be associated with delay in fine motor skills.
   C may be associated with delay in gross motor skills.
   D is often associated with cerebellar pathology.
   E is best treated by a multidisciplinary team.

15 Ipecacuanha should be given to a child with a history of having ingested

   A petrol half an hour ago.
   B ferrous sulphate 2 hours ago.
   C aspirin 6 hours ago.
   D paracetamol 6 hours ago.
   E bleach 2 hours ago.

16 The following are features of meningitis in a 9-month old baby.

    A Refusal to feed.
    B Sunken anterior fontanelle.
    C Projectile vomiting.
    D Convulsions.
    E Irritability.

17 The following statements are true of children with Turner's syndrome.

    A Hypertension is a recognised feature.
    B Increased carrying angle is characteristic.
    C Renal abnormalities are recognised associated features.
    D Most of the children have normal intellectual development.
    E They are almost invariably sterile.

18 The following statements are true of large for gestational age infants.

    A They are heavier than the 90th centile in weight for gestation.
    B They may be infants of mother with gestational diabetes.
    C They are more likely to have birth trauma.
    D They are more likely to have hypothermia.
    E They may be normal babies from large mothers.

19 The following statements are true regarding ophthalmia neonatorum.

    A This is always a benign and self-limiting condition.
    B Chloramphenicol eye drops can be prescribed without microbiological examination.
    C Infection by *Neisseria gonorrhoea* is usually acquired during vaginal delivery.
    D Systematic therapy is never required for infection by gonorrhoea.
    E Systematic therapy is never required for infection by *Chlamydia*.

20 The following are definite contraindications to pertussis immunisation.

    A Tuberous sclerosis.
    B Definite convulsion 36 hours after immunisation.
    C Infants taking corticosteroids.
    D Cystic fibrosis.
    E Prematurity.

21 An average 6-month old baby can

    A be pulled to sit with no head lag.
    B stand holding onto furniture.
    C play 'pat-a-cake'.
    D grasp an object with the palm.
    E approach an object with the index finger.

22 The following statements are true about cows' milk protein intolerance.

   A It commonly presents within the first 6 months of life.
   B It may be associated with an increased IgE level.
   C Jejunal biopsy must be performed in suspected cases.
   D Breast-fed infants are never symptomatic.
   E A dietician should be involved in the management.

23 The following statements about Hirschsprung's disease are true.

   A It may be associated with delayed passage of meconium.
   B The short-segment type is more serious than the long-segment type.
   C It may be associated with chronic constipation.
   D It may present as life-threatening illness in infancy.
   E It may be diagnosed by rectal biopsy.

24 The following statements about asthma in children are true.

   A Cough is an unusual symptom.
   B The prevalence of asthma has been decreasing in the last 20 years.
   C The severity of asthma has been decreasing in the last 20 years.
   D Children over 5 years of age are more likely to be admitted to hospital in winter months.
   E The mortality rate for childhood asthma has been declining in the last 10 years.

25 The following statements about the use of corticosteriods in asthma are true.

   A Beclomethasone may be given via a nebuliser.
   B The risk of oral candidiasis is reduced if inhaled preparations are given via a spacer device.
   C Small doses of inhaled corticosteriod may cause growth retardation.
   D Alternate day oral steroids are preferable to daily oral steroids.
   E Urine should be regularly checked for glucose if oral steroid is given continuously.

26 The following are characteristic features of cystic fibrosis.

   A Clubbing of fingers.
   B Failure to thrive.
   C Staphylococcal chest infections.
   D Steatorrhoea.
   E Diabetes mellitus.

27 Viral croup

   A is associated with inspiratory stridor.
   B is most frequently caused by respiratory syncytial virus.
   C is associated with a harsh barking cough.
   D never causes severe airway obstruction.
   E is most frequent over 4 years of age.

28 Causes of bounding pulses in infants and children include
- **A** aortic stenosis.
- **B** coarctation of the aorta.
- **C** patent ductus arteriosus.
- **D** aortic regurgitation.
- **E** congestive heart failure.

29 The following statements on congenital heart disease are correct.
- **A** The incidence is about 5 per 100 000 live births.
- **B** Acyanotic heart lesions are more common than cyanotic heart lesions.
- **C** Atrial septal defect is the most common acyanotic heart lesion.
- **D** Fallot's tetralogy and transposition of the great arteries are the two most common cyanotic heart lesions.
- **E** Acyanotic lesions generally have a better prognosis than cyanotic lesions.

30 Coarctation of the aorta
- **A** may present with sudden collapse in the first month of life.
- **B** may be asymptomatic in childhood.
- **C** may be associated with an ejection systolic murmur at the left upper sternal border.
- **D** is best detected by radio-femoral delay in the first 6 months of life.
- **E** may not require surgical correction.

31 Causes of hydrocephalus include
- **A** neural tube defects.
- **B** meningitis.
- **C** cerebral tumour.
- **D** cerebral palsy.
- **E** Down's syndrome.

32 The following are appropriate at some stage for the management of status epilepticus.
- **A** Facial oxygen.
- **B** Blood glucose check.
- **C** Intramuscular diazepam.
- **D** Intramuscular paraldehyde.
- **E** Intravenous phenytoin.

33 Appropriate drug treatments for migraine for children include
- **A** paracetamol.
- **B** aspirin.
- **C** propranolol.
- **D** pizotifen.
- **E** salbutamol.

34 Recognised causes of ataxia in children include

A Dandy–Walker syndrome
B medulloblastoma
C Chickenpox
D Guillian–Barré syndrome
E Phenytoin

35 Glandular fever in children

A is caused by Epstein–Barr virus.
B is excluded by a negative Paul–Bunnell test.
C may present with tender cervical lymphadenopathy.
D may be treated by amoxycillin.
E may be associated with splenomegaly.

36 The following statements on childhood cancer are true.

A It is the most common cause of death below 15 years of age.
B Leukaemia is the most common form of childhood cancer.
C Brain tumours are the most common solid tumours.
D Environmental factors have been demonstrated to be a major cause.
E Post-natal viral infection is a recognised cause of childhood cancer.

37 Nephrotic syndrome in children

A is usually due to membranoproliferative glomerulonephritis.
B is more common in boys.
C characteristically causes periorbital oedema initially.
D usually responds to prednisolone treatment.
E is characterised by hyperlipidaemia.

38 Causes of tall stature include

A precocious puberty.
B Marfan syndrome.
C thyrotoxicosis.
D excess growth hormone production.
E Turner's syndrome.

39 The following statements about insulin treatment are true in a child with previously diagnosed diabetes.

A Insulin should be given before meals.
B More than 50% of the total insulin should be given in the morning.
C More than 50% of the insulin should be given as short-acting insulin.
D A pen injector may be used to give long-acting insulin.
E Insulin is absorbed more rapidly if given subcutaneously in the thigh than in the abdomen.

40 Pertussis

    A seldom affects infants less than 7 months of age.
    B affects boys more than girls.
    C has an incubation period of about 7 to 14 days.
    D may cause coughing which persists for months.
    E frequently causes subconjunctival haemorrhages.

41 Congenital dislocation of the hips

    A is more common in babies with a positive family history.
    B is more common in boys than girls.
    C is more common in the right than the left hip.
    D may be diagnosed by ultrasound examination.
    E is less common in blacks.

42 Sickle-cell anaemia

    A usually presents at birth.
    B is associated with increased risk of pneumococcal infection.
    C may present with acute bone pain.
    D can cause polyuria.
    E is associated with splenomegaly in teenagers.

43 Recognised features of rickets include

    A delayed closure of the anterior fontanelle.
    B craniotabes.
    C bleeding gums.
    D genu varum.
    E cardiac failure.

44 The normal 7-month old infant

    A still has a Moro reflex.
    B can transfer objects from one hand to the other.
    C can crawl forwards.
    D can laugh.
    E can roll over from front to back.

45 Children with trisomy 21 have an increased risk of

    A hypothyroidism.
    B gastrointestinal malformations.
    C deafness.
    D Wilms tumour.
    E leukaemia.

46 Hereditary spherocytosis

  A is inherited as an autosomal recessive disorder.
  B may cause significant haemolysis in the neonatal period.
  C is more common in Mediterranean countries and the Indian Sub-continent.
  D is associated with decreased red cell osmotic fragility.
  E should be managed by splenectomy before the age of 5 years.

47 Growth hormone deficiency

  A may present as hypoglycaemia in the neonatal period.
  B is usually associated with low birth weight.
  C may cause small external genitalia in boys.
  D causes poor weight gain as well as short stature.
  E is associated with normal body proportions before puberty.

48 The following factors predispose to urinary tract infections in girls.

  A Incomplete bladder emptying.
  B Constipation.
  C Using bubble bath.
  D Obesity.
  E Myelomeningocoele.

49 Slipped upper femoral epiphysis

  A is more common in girls.
  B occurs most often between 10 and 15 years of age.
  C is rarely bilateral.
  D presents with a painless limp.
  E may result in arthritis in adult life.

50 Premature thelarche

  A usually occurs in girls aged 6 to 8 years.
  B is associated with increased growth velocity.
  C is associated with a normal final height.
  D is often associated with ovarian cyst formation.
  E is often associated with vaginal bleeding.

51 The following fractures strongly suggest child abuse.

  A Fracture of the mid-shaft of the clavicle in a 2-week old baby.
  B Metaphyseal chip fractures.
  C Epiphyseal fractures.
  D A single linear parietal fracture in a 4-year old child.
  E Rib fractures.

52 In children presenting with the nephrotic syndrome

    A microscopic haematuria indicates a poor prognosis in patients aged 2 to 6 years.

    B oral penicillin should be given if oedema and ascites are present.

    C abdominal pain may indicate hypovolaemia.

    D renal biopsy is indicated before treatment if macroscopic haematuria is present.

    E relapse occurs in 25% of patients who respond to a course of prednisolone.

53 In bronchiolitis due to respiratory syncytial virus (RSV)

    A the severity of the illness is reduced by giving intravenous hydrocortisone.

    B antibiotics should be given to prevent secondary bacterial infection.

    C the incidence of subsequent wheeze is increased in the first 2 years of life.

    D droplet spread of the infection to other children is uncommon.

    E apnoeic episodes may occur in infants.

54 Osteogenesis imperfecta

    A may be inherited as autosomal dominant or autosomal recessive.

    B is due to an abnormality in calcification.

    C may cause fractures in the perinatal period.

    D may cause short stature.

    E is often associated with hearing impairment in children.

55 *Giardia lamblia* infection in children

    A may be asymptomatic.

    B characteristically causes foul-smelling diarrhoea containing blood and mucus.

    C is more likely in immunodeficient patients.

    D may cause partial villous atrophy.

    E is easily diagnosed by finding cysts in fresh stool samples.

56 Splenomegaly is a common finding in

    A idiopathic thrombocytopenic purpura.

    B prenatally acquired HIV infection.

    C coeliac disease.

    D neonatal hepatitis.

    E Gaucher's disease.

57 In the treatment of acute idiopathic thrombocytopenic purpura,

    A bone marrow examination is essential before giving corticosteroids.

    B the platelet count recovers more quickly after corticosteroids.

    C the patient should be confined to bed until the platelet count rises to over 50×10^9/L.

    D platelet infusion is indicated when the platelet count falls below 10×10^9/L.

    E intravenous immunoglobulin may be effective.

58 The floppy infant syndrome may be due to
  A Duchenne muscular dystrophy.
  B Marfan syndrome.
  C Prader–Willi syndrome.
  D hypocalcaemia.
  E Werdnig–Hoffmann disease

59 Vitamin D deficiency
  A usually causes a normal serum calcium and a raised serum phosphate.
  B may cause genu valgum.
  C may cause pain in the legs.
  D causes generalised demineralisation of bones.
  E may cause joint swelling.

60 Meningococcal infection
  A affects mainly children aged between 3 and 12 months.
  B is usually caused by Group C meningococci in the United Kingdom.
  C can be prevented in household contacts by giving oral penicillin.
  D can be prevented by vaccination.
  E is an indication for immediate treatment with parenteral penicillin.

TEST 3
Multiple-Choice Questions

Time allowed: 2 hours
   Each question consists of an initial statement (stem) followed by five completions (items) marked A to E. Each item may be true or false, and in the examination, it is possible for the five items in any question to be all true or all false, or any intermediate combination.
   One mark (+1) will be awarded for each correct answer. One mark will be deducted (–1) for each incorrect answer. A zero (0) mark will be awarded for each 'don't know' (DK) answer.

1 The planning of child health services requires
   A collection and analysis of information regarding the population need for child health services.
   B the collaboration of providers and purchasers.
   C the collaboration of professionals from the National Health Service.
   D the planning of training programmes for professionals.
   E the involvement of managers and doctors.

2 Which of the following changes in education for children have been characteristic in the 1990s?
   A Schools are allowed more freedom to design a curriculum for children.
   B Parents are less involved in their children's education.
   C There is more awareness of bullying at school.
   D Schools are encouraged to opt out of the control of local authorities.
   E Effectiveness of schools and teaching is increasingly being monitored.

3 The following statements about foster care are true.
   A Long-term fostering is used more frequently than previously.
   B Short-term fostering can last for between 6 to 18 months.
   C Foster arrangements can only be made by local authorities.
   D Prospective foster carers may foster a maximum of four children.
   E Foster parents are given detailed information about the child's health and development.

4 The adoption panel
   A consists of between 7 to 10 members.
   B recommends whether or not the child should be freed for adoption.
   C recommends whether or not the prospective adopters would be suitable for a particular child.
   D must include a lawyer.
   E may consist of all women members.

5 The following statements about attention deficit disorder are true.

   A The condition usually develops between the ages of 6 and 9.
   B Impaired attention is necessary for the diagnosis.
   C Over-activity is necessary for the diagnosis.
   D Reading difficulty is necessary for the diagnosis.
   E It usually persists through the school years.

6 Childhood conduct disorders

   A are less common than childhood emotional disorders.
   B can be diagnosed in any 12-year old boy convicted of grievous bodily harm.
   C are more common in boys than in girls.
   D are often associated with adverse psychosocial environments.
   E include persistent school refusal.

7 Live vaccines are used to immunise against the following.

   A Tuberculosis.
   B Tetanus.
   C Whooping cough.
   D Mumps.
   E *Haemophilus influenzae* Type B.

8 Combined measles, rubella and mumps vaccine

   A is contraindicated in immunocompromised children.
   B may be given at 6 months of age.
   C may cause self-limiting aseptic meningitis.
   D may be associated with pyrexia a few days later.
   E is contraindicated in cystic fibrosis.

9 Weaning

   A should begin immediately after birth.
   B may be delayed until 1 year of age.
   C helps to replenish the baby's iron stores.
   D is a gradual process.
   E occurs at different times for different babies.

10 Phenylketonuria

   A is autosomal dominant in inheritance.
   B results from failure to convert the amino acid phenylalanine to tyrosine.
   C is detected in the neonatal period by a low tyrosine level.
   D results in mental handicap if not diagnosed early.
   E may result in neurological damage to the foetus if phenylalanine intake is not restricted in an affected pregnant woman.

11 Causes of tall stature include

A Russell–Silver syndrome.
B familial tall stature.
C Klinefelter syndrome.
D Sotos syndrome.
E intracranial tumour.

12 The average 3-year old child can

A build a tower of eight cubes.
B walk upstairs one foot per step.
C copy a circle.
D use a cup and spoon.
E stand on tip-toe.

13 Childhood squints

A are mostly caused by intraocular pathology.
B may be caused by retinoblastoma.
C sometimes cause abnormal head posture.
D are more likely to be associated with amblyopia if they are alternating.
E always require surgical correction.

14 Severe learning difficulties in children

A usually have no known cause.
B are usually associated with a relevant family history.
C are slightly more common in boys.
D may be due to Down's syndrome.
E may be associated with challenging behaviour.

15 Overdose of tricyclic antidepressants in a child may present with

A loss of consciousness.
B seizure.
C tachycardia.
D respiratory depression.
E gastrointestinal bleeding.

16 For a child with proven meningococcal septicaemia

A household contacts should be given prophylactic antibiotics.
B other children in the household may be vaccinated if the *Meningococcus* is Group B.
C blood culture may yield Gram-positive diplococci.
D there may be associated arthritis.
E adrenal haemorrhage may occur.

17 Fragile X syndrome

   A occurs in about 1 in every 1000 males.
   B is associated with small testes.
   C is associated with delayed speech development.
   D is associated with normal intelligence in 30% of those affected.
   E never occurs in females.

18 The following may occur in neonates with idiopathic respiratory distress syndrome.

   A Respiratory rate of 35 breaths per minute.
   B Expiratory grunt.
   C Sternal recession.
   D Cyanosis.
   E Air bronchogram on chest X-ray.

19 Viral infections which may be acquired from the mother prenatally include

   A rubella.
   B AIDS.
   C chickenpox.
   D cytomegalovirus.
   E toxoplasmosis.

20 The following are definite contraindications to measles immunisation.

   A Cerebral palsy.
   B Recent contact with measles.
   C Persistent coryzal symptoms.
   D Acute leukaemia.
   E Untreated tuberculosis.

21 An average 3-year old child can

   A go upstairs one foot per step.
   B copy a square.
   C kick a ball.
   D be dry day and night.
   E give own sex.

22 Cystic fibrosis

   A is autosomal recessive in inheritance.
   B affects about 1 in every 2000 live births in United Kingdom.
   C has a higher incidence in African children.
   D may result in fat-soluble vitamin deficiency.
   E gene is located on the long arm of chromosome 7.

23 Toddler diarrhoea

  A often presents with failure to thrive.
  B usually resolves spontaneously.
  C usually presents between 1 and 3 years.
  D is characterised by persistent diarrhoea.
  E is often associated with passage of undigested food.

24 The following statements about reversible airway disease in infants and children are true.

  A It is often caused by virus infection in infancy.
  B Affected children often have increased IgE level.
  C Most affected children develop symptoms by 5 years of age.
  D About 75% of the affected children have symptoms of asthma as adults.
  E The symptoms often become less severe at or before the onset of puberty.

25 Immunisation against the following infections involves live vaccines.

  A Tetanus.
  B Measles, mumps and rubella.
  C Diphtheria.
  D Pertussis.
  E *Pneumococcus.*

26 The following are important in the treatment of cystic fibrosis.

  A A low calorie intake.
  B Pancreatic enzyme supplements.
  C Vitamin C supplement.
  D Chest physiotherapy.
  E Prophylactic flucloxacillin.

27 Bronchiolitis

  A most frequently presents at 3 months of age.
  B is always caused by respiratory syncytial virus.
  C may present with poor feeding.
  D is exacerbated by cigarette smoke in the household.
  E should never be treated with more than 40% oxygen.

28 The following are symptoms and signs of heart failure in a 1-month old infant.

  A Respiratory rate of 45 breaths per minute.
  B Pulse rate of 130 per minute.
  C Liver edge 4 cm below costal margin.
  D Gallop rhythm on auscultation.
  E Poor feeding.

29 Ventricular septal defect

  A often presents at birth.
  B may present with failure to thrive.
  C may be associated with a thrill.
  D characteristically causes a pansystolic murmur at the lower left sternal border.
  E always requires surgical closure.

30 The following may be present in Fallot's tetralogy.

  A Left to right shunt.
  B Ventricular septal defect.
  C Overriding of the ventricular septum by the aorta.
  D Left ventricular hypertrophy.
  E Right ventricular hypertrophy.

31 Febrile convulsions

  A occur in about 10% of children.
  B are more frequent in those with a positive family history.
  C are more common in girls than boys.
  D frequently occur below the age of 6 months.
  E commonly occur within 24 hours of a febrile illness.

32 Complex partial seizures

  A may be secondary to cerebral tumours.
  B account for less than 10% of childhood seizures.
  C are associated with visual hallucinations.
  D are associated with learning difficulties.
  E can be treated with carbamazepine.

33 Duchenne muscular dystrophy

  A is sex linked recessive in inheritance.
  B is associated with high levels of dystrophin.
  C usually presents after the age of 5 years.
  D may be associated with mental retardation.
  E is associated with a low creatinine phosphokinase level.

34 Recognised causes of sensorineural deafness in children include

  A glue ear.
  B mumps.
  C congenital rubella syndrome.
  D elective mutism.
  E neonatal jaundice.

35 Risk factors for developing leukaemia in children include

   A Down's syndrome.
   B irradiation.
   C girls.
   D Fanconi's anaemia.
   E Cystic fibrosis.

36 The following statements about urinary tract infection in children are true.

   A In children over 1 year of age, it is more common in girls than in boys.
   B It frequently presents with urinary symptoms in infancy.
   C It only requires further investigation in children below 2 years old.
   D It is caused by *E. coli* in the majority of the cases.
   E The presence of vesico-ureteric reflux is closely related to renal scarring.

37 Recognised complications of the nephrotic syndrome include

   A pneumococcal infection.
   B venous thrombosis.
   C arterial thrombosis.
   D pleural effusion.
   E infective peritonitis.

38 Congenital hypothyroidism

   A can be screened with 100% sensitivity by the Guthrie test.
   B usually has a low TSH level.
   C requires urgent diagnosis and treatment.
   D may present with an umbilical hernia.
   E may present with prolonged jaundice in the neonatal period.

39 The following advice is appropriate for diabetic children.

   A They should take a low carbohydrate diet.
   B They should take a low saturated fat diet.
   C About 50% carbohydrate should be from highly refined sugars.
   D High fibre diet should be encouraged.
   E Rotation of injection sites should be encouraged.

40 The following statements about measles are correct.

   A It is rare under 6 months of age.
   B It is transmitted mainly by direct contact.
   C Koplik's spots appear before the rash erupts.
   D The rash is maculopapular.
   E Subacute sclerosing panencephalitis may occur 4 to 8 weeks after infection.

41 Strawberry naevi

   A are usually present from birth.
   B may increase in size in the first few months.
   C may be complicated by ulceration.
   D may be complicated by infection.
   E usually require surgical excision.

42 Beta thalassaemia major

   A usually presents between 2 and 5 years of age.
   B is usually associated with a low reticulocyte count.
   C can be diagnosed antenatally by chorionic villous biopsy.
   D usually requires regular blood transfusion.
   E should be treated with iron supplements.

43 Recognised complications of Henoch–Schönlein purpura include

   A chronic glomerulonephritis.
   B nephrotic syndrome.
   C intussusception.
   D coronary artery aneurysms.
   E gross scrotal oedema.

44 The following are common complications of anticonvulsant drugs in children.

   A Liver disease with sodium valproate.
   B Hyperactivity in young children with phenobarbitone.
   C Hirsutism with carbamazepine.
   D Increased appetite and weight gain with sodium valproate.
   E Bronchial hypersecretion with clonazepam.

45 Immunisation with combined measles, mumps and rubella vaccine (MMR vaccine) is contraindicated in

   A children with a history of urticaria after egg ingestion.
   B children with a history of vomiting after egg ingestion.
   C children with HIV infection.
   D children with atopic eczema.
   E boys with X-linked hypogammaglobulinaemia.

46 Chronic diarrhoea may be the presenting symptom in the following disorders.

   A Drinking excessive amounts of orange squash.
   B Hirschsprung's disease.
   C Hypothyroidism.
   D Immunodeficiency disorders.
   E Urinary infection.

47 Idiopathic respiratory distress syndrome

   A is associated with an increase in lung compliance.
   B is associated with pulmonary vasodilatation.
   C is often associated with right to left intrapulmonary shunting.
   D is less likely to occur in infants of heroin addicted mothers.
   E is more common in infants of diabetic mothers.

48 Conjugated hyperbilirubinaemia

   A may occur in cystic fibrosis.
   B occurs in the Crigler–Najjar syndrome.
   C occurs in breast milk jaundice.
   D may cause kernicterus.
   E may indicate biliary atresia.

49 Immunoglobulin A deficiency in children

   A occurs in approximately 1 child in 10 000.
   B is often asymptomatic.
   C is associated with an increased incidence of food allergy.
   D is associated with an increased incidence of autoimmune disease.
   E may be associated with deficiency of immunoglobulin G2.

50 Children with sickle-cell disease

   A have a chronic haemolytic anaemia.
   B often develop splenomegaly in later childhood.
   C should be immunised against *Pneumococcus* at 6 months of age.
   D have a better prognosis if the haemoglobin F level is low.
   E often develop leg ulcers.

51 Cataracts may occur in

   A galactosaemia.
   B rickets.
   C prolonged use of corticosteroids in children.
   D congenital adrenal hyperplasia.
   E congenital toxoplasmosis.

52 Human breast milk

   A is whey dominant.
   B contains specific secretory IgA.
   C contains more vitamin K than cows' milk.
   D contains more sodium than cows' milk.
   E contains primarily polyunsaturated fat.

53 Migraine in children

  A is the most common cause of headache in childhood.
  B is often associated with a positive family history.
  C is commonly associated with travel sickness.
  D may cause transient hemiparesis.
  E may be caused by eating chocolate.

54 In children presenting with acute lymphatic leukaemia, the following indicate a worse prognosis.

  A A normal white cell count.
  B Age less than 1 year.
  C Age more than 10 years.
  D Lymphadenopathy.
  E Low haemoglobin.

55 Iron deficiency may be associated with

  A gastro-oesophageal reflux.
  B thalassaemia major.
  C threadworm infestation.
  D pica.
  E drinking excessive amounts of fresh cows' milk.

56 The following changes to the circulation occur at birth.

  A Increase in pulmonary vascular resistance.
  B Increase in pulmonary blood flow.
  C Increase in systemic vascular resistance.
  D Increase in pulmonary venous return with increase in left atrial pressure.
  E Fall in cardiac output.

57 Lumbar puncture for suspected meningitis is contraindicated in the following situations.

  A Decreasing level of consciousness.
  B A child who has had a seizure lasting 40 minutes.
  C Treatment with antibiotics before admission to hospital.
  D The child with poor peripheral perfusion and a typical purpuric rash.
  E The presence of extensor plantar responses.

58 Proteinuria

  A may occur transiently in normal children during a febrile illness.
  B may occur in normal children after severe exertion.
  C may be used as a screening test for urinary infection.
  D is common in children with diurnal enuresis.
  E is often present in vesico-ureteric reflux.

59 Nocturnal enuresis
  A is often associated with stress within families.
  B occurs in 10 to 15% of 5 year olds.
  C is often associated with a family history of bed-wetting.
  D is often associated with mild daytime wetting.
  E is an indication for renal ultrasound examination.

60 Loss of consciousness may occur in
  A simple partial seizures.
  B breath holding attacks.
  C benign paroxysmal vertigo.
  D Fallot's tetralogy.
  E hyperventilation.

TEST 4
Multiple-Choice Questions

Time allowed: 2 hours

Each question consists of an initial statement (stem) followed by five completions (items) marked A to E. Each item may be true or false, and in the examination, it is possible for the five items in any question to be all true or all false, or any intermediate combination.

One mark (+1) will be awarded for each correct answer. One mark will be deducted (−1) for each incorrect answer. A zero mark will be awarded for each 'don't know' (DK) answer.

1 Health visitors

    A are involved in children's care up to the age of 10.
    B are involved in child protection issues.
    C are involved with children only.
    D play a central role in child health surveillance.
    E take over care from the midwife from 5 days after birth.

2 Health promotion

    A should be mainly carried out at the national level.
    B is achieved if the population acquires increased knowledge about health.
    C is best achieved by exaggerating the harmful effects of smoking and alcohol.
    D is less important than treatment of known illnesses.
    E usually results in an immediate beneficial effect in health terms.

3 The following statements about childminding are correct.

    A Childminders are required to register with social services departments.
    B Childminders should have completed a 1-year training course.
    C Childminding is suitable for children up to the age of 13.
    D The recommended childminder to child ratio is 1:3 for children under 5 years of age.
    E The recommended childminder to child ratio is 1:3 for children between 5–8 years of age.

4 The 1989 Children Act

    A is currently in force.
    B introduced the concept of parental rights.
    C clarified that the child's welfare is of paramount importance.
    D replaced 'Place of safety order' with 'Emergency protection order'.
    E emphasised that any delay in determining a question in relation to the upbringing of a child may prejudice his or her welfare.

5 The following are examples of primary prevention.

A Immunisation against *Haemophilus influenzae* Type B infection.
B Introduction of child-proof medicine containers.
C Fluoridation of water supplies.
D Use of steroid inhaler for asthmatic children.
E Distraction test at 9 months old.

6 At school entry review

A all children should be seen by the school nurse.
B all children should be seen by the school doctor.
C visual acuity should be measured for all children.
D a hearing screening test should be performed for all children.
E there should be good liaison with parents.

7 Vaccines against the following infections are toxoids.

A Rubella
B *Meningococcus* Type C
C Poliomyelitis
D Diphtheria
E Tetanus

8 Rubella vaccination

A is contraindicated in pregnancy.
B if given during the first trimester of pregnancy, should be followed by termination of pregnancy.
C need not be given to 11–13 year old girls since 1988.
D is rarely complicated by arthropathy.
E is the main tool in eradicating the congenital rubella syndrome.

9 Which of the following feeds are appropriate?

A Doorstep cows' milk for a 3-month old infant.
B Breast milk for a 10-month old infant who can chew solid food.
C Soya formula milk for infants with proven cows' milk intolerance.
D Sweetened orange drinks for 2-year old child.
E Chopped meat for 2-year old child.

10 Adolescents with constitutional growth delay

A should be treated with growth hormone.
B sometimes have a relevant positive family history.
C have a normal bone age.
D often have pubertal delay.
E often achieve normal adult height.

11 Isolated early breast development

A is termed thelarche.
B is rare.
C is usually associated with early pubic hair development.
D is usually associated with early menstruation.
E usually indicates ovarian pathology.

12 The following statements are true regarding childhood accident.

A It is the second most common cause of mortality above the age of 1 year.
B The most common fatal accidents are road traffic accidents.
C Poisoning is the second most common cause of fatal accidents.
D Road traffic accidents comprise more than 50% of all childhood accidents.
E Education of parents and children is the only method of prevention.

13 The following are at risk of having deafness.

A Children with delayed speech.
B Children with delayed motor development.
C Children with cerebral palsy.
D Children with cleft palate.
E Children with past history of meningitis.

14 The following findings in cerebrospinal fluid support the diagnosis of bacterial meningitis.

A CSF glucose 2 mmol/L and blood glucose 9 mmol/L.
B CSF protein 0.3 g/L.
C Clear CSF.
D Excess of lymphocytes.
E Presence of coccobacilli on microscopy of CSF.

15 The following conditions characteristically present with a macular rash.

A Meningococcal septicaemia.
B Measles.
C Reaction to drugs.
D Food allergy.
E Rubella.

16 Tuberculosis

A presents with cough in the majority of the childhood cases.
B causes regional lymph node enlargement in children.
C may be followed by meningitis within 1 year of the pulmonary infection.
D has a higher prevalence in countries with a high prevalence of AIDS.
E primary infection in children can be excluded by a normal chest X-ray.

17 The following diseases are autosomal dominant in inheritance.

  A Achondroplasia.
  B Albinism.
  C Neurofibromatosis.
  D Tuberous sclerosis.
  E Duchenne muscular dystrophy.

18 The following are associated with failure to pass meconium within 24 hours after birth.

  A Prematurity.
  B Cystic fibrosis.
  C Hirschsprung's disease.
  D Coeliac disease.
  E Lactose intolerance.

19 Breast-fed infants, compared with bottle-fed infants, are less likely to have

  A jaundice.
  B infection.
  C cows' milk intolerance.
  D atopic eczema.
  E G6PD deficiency.

20 Klinefelter's syndrome

  A is associated with karyotype XYY.
  B is associated with short stature.
  C is associated with low fertility.
  D has an incidence of about 1 in 10 000 live births.
  E is associated with small testes.

21 Causes of vomiting in the first week of life include

  A duodenal atresia.
  B pyloric stenosis.
  C coeliac disease.
  D infection.
  E appendicitis.

22 Clinical features of cystic fibrosis include

  A meconium ileus.
  B rectal prolapse.
  C short stature.
  D bronchiectasis
  E pancreatic insufficiency.

23 The following are risk factors for non-organic failure to thrive.
   A Parental unemployment.
   B Single parent.
   C Parental alcohol abuse.
   D Siblings with non-accidental injury.
   E Parental mental illness.

24 The following factors are potential trigger factors for asthma.
   A Allergens.
   B Virus infection.
   C Exercise.
   D Emotional disturbance.
   E Colouring agents such as tartrazine.

25 The following physical signs indicate that an asthma attack in a 7-year old is severe.
   A Inability to talk.
   B Cyanosis.
   C Loud wheeze.
   D Use of accessory muscles of respiration.
   E Pulsus paradoxus of 5 mmHg.

26 The following statements about acute otitis media are true.
   A It often follows a viral upper respiratory infection.
   B It may be complicated by meningitis.
   C It should be treated with benzylpenicillin.
   D Decongestants are essential.
   E Temporary hearing loss may occur.

27 Recognised causes of pneumonia in children include
   A *Pneumococcus.*
   B *Chlamydia.*
   C *Mycoplasma.*
   D *Haemophilus influenzae.*
   E *Staphylococcus.*

28 The following statements about cyanosis in infants are correct.
   A It can be more readily detected if the infant is anaemic.
   B If it is not detected clinically, the infant is well oxygenated.
   C It is often accompanied by clubbing of the fingers in the first 4 months of life in the presence of congenital heart disease.
   D It is readily reversed by placing the infant in 100% oxygen if cyanosis is caused by congenital heart disease.
   E It is always present from birth in transposition of the great arteries.

29 Atrial septal defect

    A is more likely to be complicated by bacterial endocarditis than ventricular septal defect.

    B is characteristically associated with wide splitting of the second heart sound.

    C often presents at birth.

    D characteristically presents with heart failure.

    E is characteristically associated with a soft ejection murmur at the left upper sternal border.

30 Hypercyanotic attacks associated with Fallot's tetralogy

    A are rarely fatal.

    B may be triggered by exertion.

    C may be associated with loss of consciousness.

    D should be managed by placing the child in a knee-elbow position in 100% oxygen.

    E may be prevented and treated with propranolol.

31 Febrile convulsions

    A may follow pertussis immunisation.

    B may follow measles immunisation.

    C often last more than 15 minutes.

    D are most frequently caused by bacterial infection.

    E are always bilateral.

32 Sodium valproate

    A is effective in treating absence attacks (petit mal).

    B is effective in treating generalised tonic-clonic epilepsy (grand mal).

    C may cause alopecia.

    D can cause fatal hepatic toxicity.

    E should be taken before meals.

33 Duchenne muscular dystrophy

    A can be diagnosed on the basis of EMG features.

    B can be diagnosed by muscle biopsy.

    C can be diagnosed antenatally.

    D can cause cardiomyopathy.

    E often results in scoliosis.

34 Children with infantile autism

    A first show symptoms between 3 and 5 years of age.

    B characteristically have delusions.

    C have gross deficits in speech development.

    D may exhibit stereotyped movements.

    E respond normally to their own parents.

35 Presenting symptoms of leukaemia may include

A lethargy.
B anorexia.
C easy bruising.
D unusually serious infection.
E bone pain.

36 The following statements about treatment and prevention of urinary tract infection are true.

A Amoxycillin is the antibiotic of first choice.
B Co-trimoxazole has fewer side-effects than trimethoprim.
C Trimethoprim can be given for prophylaxis.
D Prophylactic treatment can be given once daily in the morning.
E Failure to respond clinically within 48 hours generally implies that the organism is resistant to the antibiotic.

37 Causes of precocious puberty include

A adrenal hyperplasia.
B Turner's syndrome.
C intracranial tumours.
D haematocolpos.
E granulosa cell ovarian tumour.

38 Recognised causes of rickets include

A coeliac disease.
B dietary deficiency.
C sarcoidosis.
D chronic renal failure.
E osteogenesis imperfecta.

39 Complications of meningitis include

A conductive deafness.
B hydrocephalus.
C subdural collection of fluid.
D epilepsy.
E cerebral palsy.

40 Erythema infectiosum

A is caused by parainfluenza virus.
B may cause pruritus.
C may cause lymphadenopathy.
D is also known as sixth disease.
E may cause stillbirth if pregnant mothers are infected.

41 Anorexia nervosa

    A occurs in males in about 5% of cases.
    B is characterised by distortion of body image.
    C may be associated with hypokalaemia.
    D may be associated with laxative abuse.
    E may be treated by a combination of individual and family therapy.

42 Breath-holding attacks

    A usually present after the age of 5 years.
    B may be precipitated by minor emotional upset.
    C are never associated with loss of consciousness.
    D are followed by rapid recovery.
    E should be treated with prophylactic anticonvulsants if occurring frequently.

43 Diaphragmatic hernia

    A occurs most often on the right side.
    B occurs through the foramen of Morgagni in most cases.
    C can be diagnosed antenatally.
    D is usually accompanied by lung hypoplasia on the affected side.
    E may be accompanied by persistent fetal circulation.

44 Von Willebrand's disease in children

    A is inherited as an autosomal recessive disorder.
    B may be asymptomatic.
    C may present with recurrent epistaxis.
    D can always be diagnosed at birth by blood tests.
    E commonly presents with bleeding from the umbilical cord.

45 Recurrent abdominal pain in children

    A affects 10% of children over the age of 5 years.
    B most often occurs in the right lower quadrant of the abdomen.
    C is associated with organic pathology in about 45% of cases.
    D is likely to be related to food allergy if it occurs at meal times.
    E is often associated with headache.

46 The incidence of the following is increased in the children of parents who smoke.

    A Pneumonia in infancy.
    B Glue ears.
    C Sudden infant death syndrome.
    D Hospital admissions due to asthma.
    E Recurrent wheeze in infancy.

47 Hair loss in children may be due to

   A sodium valproate.
   B phenytoin.
   C hair pulling by the child.
   D scalp ringworm.
   E wearing a ponytail.

48 Meningism may occur in

   A pneumonia.
   B bronchiolitis.
   C tonsillitis.
   D Reye's syndrome.
   E migraine.

49 Congestive cardiac failure in infants

   A is most often caused by left-sided obstructive lesions.
   B often occurs in Fallot's tetralogy.
   C frequently causes failure to thrive.
   D commonly causes vomiting.
   E often causes sweating.

50 In infants born to heroin addicted mothers

   A there is an increased incidence of hyaline membrane disease.
   B administration of naloxone at birth is indicated.
   C irritability is the most common symptom.
   D phenobarbitone is widely used to control many of the symptoms.
   E the incidence of sudden infant death syndrome is increased.

51 Acute epiglottitis

   A is caused by parainfluenza virus.
   B is associated with septicaemia.
   C responds to intravenous steroids.
   D requires elective endotracheal intubation.
   E is associated with drooling and difficulty in swallowing.

52 Hypoglycaemia in children may occur

   A in growth hormone deficiency.
   B in liver disease.
   C following a prolonged seizure.
   D in congenital adrenal hyperplasia.
   E in medium chain acyl dehydrogenase (MCAD) deficiency.

53 Painful joints may occur in

A Henoch–Schönlein purpura.
B idiopathic thrombocytopenic purpura.
C acute leukaemia.
D sickle-cell disease.
E thalassaemia intermedia.

54 Perthes' disease

A affects the proximal femoral epiphysis of the femur.
B is more common in girls.
C may be bilateral in a few patients.
D most often presents with a limp.
E may result in premature osteoarthritis of the hip.

55 The following conditions have autosomal dominant inheritance.

A Tuberous sclerosis
B Christmas disease
C Congenital spherocytosis
D Ataxia telangiectasia
E Pierre Robin syndrome

56 Neuroblastoma

A is the most common solid tumour of childhood.
B often presents with haematuria.
C is often associated with metastases at the time of initial presentation.
D may present as an incidental finding on chest X-ray.
E has a better prognosis than Wilms' tumour.

57 Chickenpox

A is caused by a RNA virus.
B usually has a prodromal period with fever and upper respiratory symptoms lasting 3 or 4 days.
C has an incubation period of 5 days.
D may cause severe illness in the infant if it is acquired in pregnancy.
E may be complicated by acute cerebellar ataxia.

58 Wheeze may occur in

A infection due to *Mycoplasma pneumoniae*.
B pulmonary tuberculosis in children.
C adenovirus infection.
D bronchopulmonary dysplasia.
E gastro-oesophageal reflux.

59 Severe learning difficulty

  A is more common in girls.
  B is often associated with behaviour problems.
  C is very common in boys with Duchenne muscular dystrophy.
  D occurs in the fragile X syndrome.
  E is common in Turner's syndrome.

60 Vesicoureteric reflux

  A is present in 10% of children with urinary infection.
  B causes loin pain.
  C may be transient after bladder infection.
  D is associated with renal scarring in 5% of cases.
  E is usually detected by renal ultrasound scan.

TEST 5
Multiple-Choice Questions

Time allowed: 2 hours
Each question consists of an initial statement (stem) followed by five completions (items) marked A to E. Each item may be true or false, and in the examination, it is possible for the five items in any question to be all true or all false, or any intermediate combination.
One mark (+1) will be awarded for each correct answer. One mark will be deducted (–1) for each incorrect answer. A zero (0) mark will be awarded for each 'don't know' (DK) answer.

1 The following statements are true regarding education.

A The statutory school age is between 5 and 16 years.
B Local authorities have a statutory requirement to provide education to children between the ages of 3 and 5 years.
C Pupils are admitted to secondary school at the age of 10 years.
D Parents are by law required to send their children to school at statutory school age.
E Education between the ages of 16 and 18 is always provided either in a sixth-form or a sixth form college.

2 Health education

A should be taught as a separate subject in schools.
B is outside the National Curriculum.
C must be taught by biology teachers.
D need not be provided after 14 years of age.
E includes substance use and misuse.

3 The following statements about children under the care of local authorities are true.

A The number has increased in the last decade.
B The use of residential homes has been reduced in favour of foster care.
C Children from families receiving income support have a higher chance of being in care.
D Asian children have a higher chance of being in care.
E Afro-Caribbean children have a higher chance of being in care.

4 An Education Supervision Order

   A may be made on a 17-year old child.
   B is usually made only if the school attendance of a child is unsatisfactory.
   C places the child under the supervision of a local education authority.
   D usually lasts until the child reaches majority.
   E excludes the parents from taking further decisions relating to the education of the child.

5 Which of the following statements are true regarding child health surveillance?

   A Innovative screening tests are the most important.
   B The paediatrician is the main health professional for pre-school children.
   C The school nurse plays an important role for children of school age.
   D Parents should always be closely involved.
   E The child health clinic plays an important part in the delivery of child health surveillance.

6 Colour vision

   A should be tested before children leave school.
   B defects can be treated.
   C testing by Ishihara charts is very sensitive.
   D testing by Ishihara charts allows detailed career guidance.
   E testing is usually unnecessary for boys.

7 Vaccines against the following infections are usually given between 2 and 9 months of age.

   A Diphtheria
   B Mumps
   C Rubella
   D Poliomyelitis
   E *Haemophilus influenzae* Type B

8 Whooping cough

   A is universally caused by *Bordetella pertussis*.
   B may cause apnoea attacks in babies.
   C has the worst prognosis in children aged between 3 and 5 years.
   D never occurs in children who have received the full course of whooping cough vaccination.
   E symptoms usually resolve by 2 weeks.

9 Cows' milk intolerance

   A is a common cause of wheezing in infants.
   B may occur with total breast-feeding.
   C may cause anaemia.
   D may be treated with hydrolysed protein formulae.
   E diagnosed in infancy implies the child must avoid milk products until adolescence.

10 The following statements are true about Turner's syndrome.

    A It affects 1 in every 600 live births.
    B It may cause oedema of the hands and feet in the newborn period.
    C High-dose human growth hormone may increase final adult height.
    D It may present with primary amennorhoea.
    E It may be associated with coarctation of the aorta.

11 The following findings should arouse concern.

    A Presence of the Moro reflex at 12 months of age.
    B Asymmetrical Moro reflex at 5 months of age.
    C Presence of the stepping reflex at 3 months of age.
    D Asymmetrical tonic neck reflex at 12 months of age.
    E The parachute reaction at 12 months of age.

12 The following statements are true regarding the rate of childhood accidents.

    A Reduction is one of the key targets in the 'Health of the Nation'.
    B The accident rate is highest in social class V.
    C Legislation has an important role in prevention.
    D The primary care team has an important role in prevention.
    E Boys have a higher rate of accidental head injury than girls.

13 The following may be features of separation anxiety disorder.

    A Irrational preoccupying worry that harm might befall the child's mother.
    B Irrational excessive fear of dogs.
    C Persistent refusal to go to sleep without being next to the child's parents.
    D Repeated nightmares about the theme of separation from the child's parents.
    E Irrational fear and avoidance of strangers.

14 Sudden infant death syndrome

    A is more common in males than females.
    B occurs in less than 1 in 500 live births.
    C is more common in lower social classes.
    D is more common in babies nursed in the prone position.
    E is more common in summer.

15 The following are recognised complications of chickenpox.

    A Cerebellar ataxia.
    B Pneumonia.
    C Subacute sclerosing panencephalitis.
    D Koplik's spots.
    E Cold sores.

16 The following statements are true regarding the Mantoux test.

A It is given intradermally.
B In normal clinical practice, 100 TU (tuberculin unit) are initially used.
C The test should be read 24 hours after administration.
D The result is indicated by the area of erythema.
E It is usually administered on the upper third of the extensor surface of the arm.

17 The following diseases are sex-linked in inheritance.

A G6PD deficiency.
B Haemophilia B (Christmas Disease).
C Galactosaemia.
D Congenital spherocytosis.
E Chronic granulomatous disease.

18 Causes of jaundice in the first 24 hours of life include

A physiological jaundice.
B ABO incompatibility.
C congenital spherocytosis.
D breast-milk jaundice.
E hypothyroidism.

19 The following statements about tic disorders are true.

A More than 5% of children have experienced transient tics.
B They are more common in girls than boys.
C They are more common in those with a positive family history.
D Repetition of certain words may be a feature.
E Repeated hissing may be a feature.

20 An average 9-month old baby can

A stand holding on to furniture.
B pick up a raisin between thumb and finger.
C creep upstairs.
D build a tower of two cubes.
E say two or three words with meaning.

21 The following statements about pyloric stenosis are true.

A It is more common in male infants.
B The incidence is increased if there is a family history of the condition.
C It characteristically develops at about 6 months of age.
D A pyloric mass may be palpable in the left upper quadrant.
E Ultrasound may help in making the diagnosis.

22 Causes of rectal bleeding in childhood include

A anal fissure.
B Henoch–Schönlein purpura.
C cows' milk intolerance.
D intussusception.
E pyloric stenosis.

23 Causes of acute stridor in a 4-year old include

A asthma.
B acute epiglottitis.
C foreign body.
D cystic fibrosis.
E pneumococcal pneumonia.

24 The following statements about drug therapy in asthma are true.

A Drugs have a more rapid action if administered by inhalation than if administered orally.
B Nebulisers deliver about 50% of the drugs to the lungs.
C The choice of drugs depend on the pattern of disease of the child.
D Side-effects of salbutamol are more troublesome if given orally than if inhaled.
E Prophylactic therapy with sodium cromoglycate or inhaled steroids is indicated if inhaled beta-agonist is required every day.

25 The following statements about the treatment of an acute asthma attack are true.

A Nebulised salbutamol should not be given if the child is taking salbutamol via an inhaler.
B Steroids should never be given if the symptoms have improved after nebulised salbutamol.
C A chest X-ray is mandatory.
D Oxygen should never be given at a concentration higher than 28%.
E Aminophylline should be administered if the child is on regular theophylline.

26 The following statements about pertussis are true.

A The most important causative organism is *Bordetella pertussis*.
B The causative organisms are usually isolated from the throat swab.
C It is often associated with a high neutrophil count at the early stages of the disease.
D The disease is more severe in infants than in older children.
E Infants may develop apnoea.

27 Foreign body inhalation in children

   A occurs more commonly in the younger age group.
   B may cause wheezing.
   C is more common in boys.
   D commonly causes impaction in the left main bronchus.
   E is an indication for bronchoscopy.

28 Causes of left to right shunt include

   A ventricular septal defect.
   B coarctation of the aorta.
   C atrial septal defect.
   D pulmonary stenosis.
   E patent ductus arteriosus.

29 Patent ductus arteriosus

   A is more common in premature infants than in full-term infants.
   B may cause heart failure in infants.
   C is associated with a low diastolic blood pressure.
   D is characteristically associated with a continuous murmur loudest at the lower left sternal edge.
   E may require surgical closure.

30 Hypertension in children

   A is always secondary to other diseases.
   B is commonly associated with obesity.
   C may be associated with a family history of hypertension.
   D should be investigated for underlying renal disease.
   E is frequently asymptomatic.

31 Absence attacks (petit mal)

   A are associated with an aura.
   B are associated with tonic-clonic jerks of the limbs.
   C are more frequent in those with a positive family history.
   D are more common in boys than girls.
   E are associated with a characteristic EEG pattern.

32 Phenytoin

   A is effective in treating complex partial seizures (temporal lobe epilepsy).
   B is effective in treating petit mal.
   C can be given as twice daily dosage.
   D may cause ataxia.
   E may cause gum hyperplasia.

33 Cerebral palsy

    A is a progressive condition.
    B is caused by birth trauma in the majority of the cases.
    C may be caused by tuberous sclerosis.
    D has an incidence of less than 1% of all live births.
    E may be due to hyperbilirubinaemia in the neonatal period.

34 Recognised features of neurofibromatosis include

    A café-au-lait spots.
    B adenoma sebaceum.
    C scoliosis.
    D deafness.
    E renal artery stenosis.

35 Idiopathic thrombocytopenic purpura

    A has a Mendelian inheritance.
    B usually presents between 5 and 10 years of age.
    C usually remits spontaneously with no treatment.
    D is associated with a low neutrophil count.
    E may be treated with a course of prednisolone.

36 Vesico-ureteric reflux

    A is usually congenital in origin.
    B usually persists until adulthood without surgical treatment.
    C may be demonstrated by micturating cystourethrogram.
    D occurs in less than 10% of children with urinary tract infection.
    E can be graded depending on dilatation of the ureters, calyces and renal pelvis.

37 Causes of secondary amenorrhoea include

    A polycystic ovarian syndrome.
    B stress.
    C weight loss.
    D Turner's syndrome.
    E uterine fibroids.

38 Features of congenital adrenal hyperplasia in girls include

    A ambiguous genitalia.
    B hypertension.
    C abnormal pigmented genitalia.
    D hirsuitism.
    E striae.

39 Gastroenteritis in children

   A is usually caused by *E. coli.*
   B is more common in breast-fed infants than bottle-fed infants.
   C may result in metabolic acidosis.
   D occurs mainly in children over 2 years of age.
   E may cause convulsions.

40 Chickenpox

   A has an incubation period of between 7 to 14 days.
   B has a high mortality rate in babies of mothers infected less than a week before delivery.
   C may be complicated by Reye's syndrome.
   D may be treated with acyclovir in immunocompromised children.
   E may be associated with vesicles on the mucous membrane of the inside of the mouth.

41 Recognised causes of plagiocephaly include

   A sternomastoid tumour
   B craniosynostosis
   C positioning
   D congenital rubella syndrome
   E Down's syndrome.

42 The following features suggest truancy rather than school refusal.

   A The child complains of abdominal pain.
   B The child has a good academic record.
   C The child is 8 years old.
   D The child has antisocial behaviour.
   E The parents are unaware of the child's absence from school.

43 Haemorrhagic disease of the newborn

   A usually presents with umbilical bleeding on the first day of life.
   B occurs mainly in breast-fed babies.
   C commonly causes massive pulmonary haemorrhage.
   D may present with haematemesis and melaena.
   E can be prevented by intramuscular vitamin K at birth.

44 Ostium secundum atrial septal defect

   A often occurs in children with Trisomy 21.
   B is generally asymptomatic in children.
   C causes fixed splitting of the first heart sound.
   D is associated with a systolic murmur due to flow across the atrial septal defect.
   E is the most common heart defect to be complicated by bacterial endocarditis.

45 Macroglossia may occur in
  A congenital hypothyroidism.
  B Beckwith–Wiedemann's syndrome.
  C Down's syndrome.
  D Turner's syndrome.
  E glycogen storage disease.

46 The following are recognised associations.
  A Turner's syndrome and pulmonary stenosis.
  B Down's syndrome and atrioventricular canal defects.
  C Noonan's syndrome and coarctation of the aorta.
  D Tuberous sclerosis and cardiac rhabdomyomata.
  E Marfan's syndrome and mitral regurgitation.

47 Homozygous beta thalassaemia
  A is associated with a low haemoglobin at birth.
  B can be diagnosed antenatally at 12 weeks gestation.
  C always requires treatment with regular blood transfusions.
  D may result in delayed onset of puberty.
  E may be successfully treated with a bone marrow transplant.

48 Syncope in children
  A occurs suddenly without preceding symptoms.
  B is accompanied by a weak or impalpable peripheral pulse.
  C may result in muscle jerking.
  D may be followed by urinary incontinence.
  E should be managed by a trial of anticonvulsants if occurring frequently.

49 Childhood absence epilepsy (petit mal)
  A usually begins before the age of 5 years.
  B is often associated with learning difficulties.
  C is accompanied by a 3 per second spike and wave activity on EEG.
  D responds well to treatment with carbamazepine.
  E usually has a good prognosis.

50 Specific reading disorder (developmental dyslexia)
  A may be due to inadequate schooling.
  B is often associated with spelling difficulties.
  C may be associated with poor oral reading skills.
  D is commonly associated with developmental speech delay.
  E is often associated with a low IQ.

51 Inheritance of the following conditions is X linked.

   A Von Willebrand's disease.
   B Huntington's chorea.
   C Wiskott–Aldrich syndrome.
   D Duchenne muscular dystrophy.
   E Achondroplasia.

52 Plagiocephaly

   A is usually associated with craniosynostosis.
   B may be associated with thoracic asymmetry.
   C is associated with a preference to look to one side.
   D is associated with abnormalities on cranial CT scan.
   E has a good prognosis.

53 The following drugs may be teratogenic if taken in pregnancy.

   A Penicillin.
   B Sodium valproate.
   C Phenytoin.
   D Warfarin.
   E Heparin.

54 Cystic fibrosis

   A affects 1 child in every 10 000.
   B may be diagnosed antenatally using chorion villous biopsy.
   C may present with nasal polyposis.
   D is diagnosed when a sweat chloride of more than 70 mmol/L is found in 50 mg sweat.
   E should be treated with a high protein low fat diet.

55 The incidence of sudden infant death syndrome is increased in

   A summer.
   B babies of Asian families.
   C babies of mothers who are less than 20 years of age.
   D babies who sleep in the supine position.
   E babies whose mothers smoked during pregnancy.

56 Congenital adrenal hyperplasia due to 21-hydroxylase deficiency may present with

   A ambiguous genitalia in male infants.
   B a salt-losing crisis during the first 48 hours of life.
   C precocious puberty in males.
   D delayed menarche.
   E hypertension.

57 Fetal haemoglobin

    A comprises 40% of haemoglobin at birth.
    B consists of 2 alpha and 2 delta chains.
    C has a lower affinity for oxygen than adult haemoglobin.
    D falls to less than 2% total haemoglobin at age 1 year.
    E declines more rapidly after birth in children with beta thalassaemia and sickle-cell disease.

58 The normal 3-year old child

    A can copy a circle.
    B can stand on one leg for 10 seconds.
    C can build a tower of nine cubes.
    D can draw a man with a head, trunk and four limbs.
    E can cut with a pair of scissors.

59 Pertussis

    A may present with apnoeic attacks in infants.
    B is most infective about 1 week after bouts of paroxysmal coughing have started.
    C is often associated with fever.
    D may be associated with coughing lasting for several months.
    E is often associated with a normal chest X-ray.

60 Acquired hypothyroidism in children

    A is most often due to autoimmune thyroiditis in the United Kingdom.
    B may present with isolated breast development in girls.
    C may present with large testes and short stature in boys.
    D often results in permanent intellectual deficits.
    E is more common in children with Down's syndrome.

ADVICE ON THE CLINICAL SECTION

General

In the long case, you have only 40 minutes with the patient and 20 minutes to present it and be questioned by the examiners. Therefore, you must elicit the essential points in the history and perform an examination efficiently. The best way to prepare for this is to frequently practise seeing patients within this time limit and present the case to your seniors.

Equipment

While the examination centre will provide all necessary equipment, it is advisable to bring your own equipment for two reasons. Firstly, it will save time looking or asking for the equipment. Secondly, it is an advantage to use a familiar piece of equipment. This is especially true for equipment used for developmental assessment. If you are familiar with the developmental milestones related to 1 inch cubes, you do not want to use other equipment to test for fine motor development.

You may wish to bring the following:

- Paediatric stethoscope.
- Paediatric patella hammer.
- Pen torch.
- Three 1-inch cubes.
- Pen and paper.
- Eye occluder.
- A toy (e.g. car).
- Measuring tape (which can also be used as a dangling object).
- Small objects (e.g. raisins or 'hundreds and thousands').

Hints on the long case

In the long case, it is important to take a good history, not only of physical symptoms, but also of social, behavioural and educational aspects. Growth assessment is also important.

While it is important to be adept at paediatric history taking and examination, it may prove impossible to complete a full history and examination on all the physical, social, behavioural and psychiatric, growth and developmental aspects within the time constraints of the examination. It is therefore essential to give priority to those areas which are relevant to that particular case. However, you should always take a brief history on all these aspects.

Meeting the patient and the parents

- You will see the patient and the parents on your own without the examiners.
- Introduce yourself to the parents, explaining you are taking an examination. Find out the main problems in the first two minutes. Then decide whether a detailed history relating to the educational, social development and psychological aspects is important for the particular child. Generally speaking, a detailed history of the physical aspects is nearly always needed.
- You will normally examine the child after history taking. However, you may sometimes want to be opportunistic in your physical examination (e.g. listen to the child's heart when he is still asleep and you know from the history that he has cardiology problems.)
- Go through the essential points relevant to the presenting symptoms first; ask about other points afterwards if you have time.
- Always ask about
    — brief birth history;
    — immunisation;
    — current medication and treatment;
    — brief social history; and
    — other professionals involved.
- Physical examination
    — Observe the child while you are taking the history. Much information (especially developmental assessment and mental state assessment) can be gained by observation alone.
    — Examine the relevant system first while you still have the child's cooperation.
    — Always plot height and weight on appropriate charts (the measurements are given to you),
    — Measure the blood pressure (the measurement may also be given to you)
    — The posture or gait of the child is more important than testing the power and reflexes in neurological examination.
    — Always test the urine (the sample is given to you).
- At the end, always ask the parents
    — what the diagnosis is. (Most parents will tell you. If they reply 'It is for you to find out', take it gracefully.)
    — Are there any other questions I should have asked?
- Allow at least 10 minutes at the end to
    — clarify any points with the parents;
    — prepare a summary of the case;
    — prepare a differential diagnosis, and
    — prepare a management strategy.

Meeting the examiners

- Listen carefully to the examiners' first instruction. They may ask you to 'Tell us about the case', 'Tell us about the case briefly' or 'Give us a summary of the case'. Do as you are told.

- You should have written a two to three sentence summary of the case before meeting the examiners. You will need this either at the beginning or the end of your presentation. Include the educational and social aspects if they are important to the case.
- You have less than 10 minutes to present the case. You should be concise and mention only the positive and important negative points. For example, 'His immunisation is up to date,' is sufficient without listing all the immunisations the child has received. If the developmental history of a child is normal, just give one most recent milestone for each of the four areas (gross motor, fine motor, language, social).
- When you are asked about the differential diagnosis, give the most likely diagnosis first.

General format of a paediatric history

Name: *Age:*   *Sex:*

Presenting problems

Systematic questions

These can be covered briefly, focusing on points which may be relevant.

Past medical history

This includes:

- birth history – Birth weight, gestation, how delivered, condition at birth, neonatal treatment;
- feeding history (for infants and toddlers) – Bottle or breast, amount of feed, time of weaning;
- immunisation history.

Drugs and allergy

Family history

Social history

- parents (age, occupation, smoking habit), siblings (age);
- schooling (type of school (normal or special needs)), academic progress, relationship with other students and teachers);
- behavioural – problems with sleep, tantrums, school refusal, truant etc.
- housing – number of rooms, special problems etc.

Developmental history

- Parental concerns with hearing and vision.
- Developmental milestones in all four areas.

Physical examination

- Plot the child's height, weight and head circumference on the appropriate charts.
- Observe the general behaviour of the child and his relationship with parents
- Examine the relevant systems as appropriate.
- Perform a detailed developmental assessment if there is a suggestion of developmental delay in the history.
- Measure BP and test urine.

Assessment of visual function

If the child is suspected to have visual problems affecting his education, the following should be considered:

- distant visual acuity (use the Sheridan–Gardner test if the child is more than 3–4 years old; use the Snellen chart if the child is more than about 8 years old);
- near visual acuity – important for education purposes;
- visual fields – important for education purposes;
- colour vision – use Ishihara charts;
- cause and progression – the cause for the visual problem and whether determination is likely;
- examine the eyes for symmetry, external eye abnormalities, red reflex and fundoscopy.

Short cases

This part lasts for 30 minutes of which 10 minutes will be devoted to developmental testing, including testing hearing or vision.

Section 1 (a) Testing hearing or vision and (b) developmental assessment

Testing hearing

You may be asked to perform the distraction test for a 7–8-month old child.

- Close the door and ensure the room is quiet.
- Stand behind the child.
- Check that you do not form a shadow as a cue for the child.
- Ask the mother to sit the child on her lap, and not to react to sound.
- Ask one examiner to be the distractor, and capture the child's attention (e.g. with a toy). The distractor should not establish eye contact with the child.
- Ask the other examiner to stand outside the child's field of vision!
- A warbler device will probably be available. It is held at 50 cm from the child's ear and at the same level. It is wise to familiarise youself with this device before the examination.
- If a warbler device is not available, use a Manchester rattle held at 1 m from the child, or 'S' voice, but make sure it is of minimal intensity (high frequency), and a minimal 'M' voice for low frequency.

- Produce test sounds when the child's attention is held by the examiner.
- A positive response is localisation of the sound by the child turning his or her head.
- Praise the child if he or she locates the sound.
- Repeat the test twice. A correct response in at least two out of three trials constitutes a pass in the hearing test.

Testing vision

- Ask about parental concerns regarding vision or squint.
- Eye movement – whether there is restriction of eye movements.
- Shine light with the pen torch from a distance and note the symmetry of corneal reflex.
- Perform cover test to detect squint.

Visual acuity (distant)

— Infant: As a rough assessment determine whether the child is able to follow a dangling object placed about 30 cm in front of him or her.
— Age 3–7: STYCAR letter test – matching capital letters presented at 3 m with the same letters on a key card in a different order. There are three types of key cards:
    five capital letters – for child about 3 years old.
    seven capital letters – for child about 4 years old.
    nine capital letters – for child above 5 years old.
— Age above 8: Use the Snellen Chart as in an adult.

Visual acuity (near)

— Use 'hundreds and thousands' and observe the size of sweets the child is able to locate.

Developmental assessment

- Choose a set of developmental tests spread over the whole age range to 5 years, ensuring all four areas (gross motor, fine motor, language and social) are covered, and using a minimal set of equipment.
- Develop a routine of testing children in each area of development, so that the tests follow on smoothly. Start with the tests which most easily give you the attention of the child.
- Examples are:

— 6 months or less. Dangle object in front of the child. Observe the ability of the child to follow the object with his or her eyes horizontally, vertically and in circles.
The child may try to grasp the object automatically. Observe the nature of the grasp, the ability to transfer to the other hand, ability to hold two objects in one hand etc.
Offer the child a small object (e.g. a raisin). Observe the child's approach.

Listen for the sound he or she produces.

Head control from supine and other positions.

— *Between 6 months and 1 year old*. Offer the child a 1-inch brick. Observe whether he or she can reach out and transfer the brick to the other hand. Offer another 1-inch brick. Observe whether he can bring them together or whether he can hold them both together in one hand.
Offer the child a small object (e.g. a raisin). Determine the visual function and nature of grasp (pincer or palmer grasp).

Listen to the sound the child makes.

Try playing pat-a-cake, get the child to wave goodbye (for a child of almost 1 year old), object permanence.

— *Between 1 and 3 years old*: Offer some 1-inch bricks. Observe the child's ability to build towers, gates etc.

Offer a pen and pencil. Observe the child's ability to copy or imitate horizontal or vertical lines, circle.

Listen for the language the child produces. (e.g. word phrases etc.)

Test for understanding (e.g. ask his name, sex, etc.)

Ability to walk with or without hand held. Stand on one foot, try stairs.

- Try to limit the developmental age in each of the four areas as you are assessing. For example, if you have established that a child can sit unsupported, you know that the gross motor developmental age is at least 9 months. You should then test for items with a developmental age above, not below, 9 months.
- When you present your findings, present each of the four areas of development separately. Explain how you arrive at your estimated developmental age in that area by giving a milestone the child has achieved and one he or she has not. Then give your general conclusion. An example is as follows.

He can sit unsupported momentarily, but he cannot sit unsupported with pivot. Therefore, his gross motor developmental age is about 9 months. He can pick up a small object between the finger and thumb, but he does not yet have a mature pincer grasp. Therefore, his fine motor developmental age is also about 9 months. He combines syllables, for example, by saying 'da da', but he has not said a word with meaning. Hence, his language development is also consistent with 9 months. He shows stranger anxiety. He has not yet developed object permanence. Hence, his social development is also consistent with 9 months.

As his chronological age is 18 months, he appears to have global developmental delay.

Candidates often get disheartened by the long lists of developmental milestones to be remembered. Many try to learn them all, only to get hopelessly confused. The key lies in making up a shortlist of the milestones that seem natural to you, spread evenly between the four main areas of development and age groups. You should then learn the shortlist thoroughly so that you can easily recall them. Table 1 shows an example of this shortlist.

Section 2 – short cases

The main purpose of this section is to assess your ability to recognise abnormal physical signs. Below are some common short cases:

Congenital heart disease ('Examine the heart') (see Fig. 1)

• Look for cyanosis or clubbing.
• Palpate brachial pulse for volume.
• Look for radio-femoral delay (i.e. coarctation of aorta).
• Inspect chest for abnormal shape or previous surgical scars.
• Perform palpation for apex beat, thrill, or heave.
• Listen to lower left sternal edge, apex, aortic and pulmonary areas, and over carotids.
• Describe second heart sound (e.g. loud P2, fixed splitting of second heart sound etc.).
• For murmurs, describe:
  — Systolic or diastolic.
  — If systolic, whether pansystolic or ejection systolic. If diastolic, which part of diastole?
  — Where loudest?
  — Intensity (grade between 1 – 6) of the murmur.
  — Radiation.
• Signs of heart failure (e.g. tachypnoea, crepitations, enlarged liver).
• Ask the examiner for the child's blood pressure.

Respiratory system

Chronic asthma and cystic fibrosis are the most likely conditions to appear in short cases.

You should listen carefully to the examiner's instruction. If the instruction is *'Listen to the chest'*, you should just listen to the chest. The following guide assumes that the instruction is *'Examine the respiratory system'.*

(a) General:

• Clubbing – This is important to distinguish between asthma (no clubbing) and cystic fibrosis (with clubbing).
• Cyanosis – Compare the colour of the lips or tongue of the child with a normal adult (e.g. the examiner).
• Comfort – Can the child speak in sentences, phrases or single words only due to breathing difficulties?

Table 1 Developmental assessment (a deliberately restricted list that can be demonstrated in exam situations).

Age	Gross motor	Fine motor	Social	Language
6 weeks	Lifts head 45° in prone position	Follows dangling object past the midline	Smiles at mother	Vocalises laugh
4 months	Minimal head lag when pulled to sitting position	Reaches out for objects Follows objects through 180°		
6 months	Sits with support	Palmar grasp of toys, which are put to mouth	Interested	Turns to voice Imitates speech voice
9 months	Sits unsupported	Thumb–finger grasp	Starts stranger anxiety Imitates hand clapping	Babbles loudly e.g. dad-dad Responds to distraction (see below)
1 year	Walks with a hand held Stands alone momentarily	Index and pincer grasp	Object permanence Waves goodbye	1–2 words with meaning Understands simple commands
18 months	Walks alone steadily	Tower of three cubes Scribbles	Drinks from a cup	5–20 recognisable words
2 years	Runs, walks up and often down stairs two feet per step	Tower of six cubes Vertical and horizontal lines	Uses a spoon	Two-word phrases Says more than 40 words
3 years	Walks upstairs one foot per step	Imitates a bridge and can copy a circle	Dresses with help	Talks in sentences Can give own name
4 years	Walks downstairs one foot per step	Builds a step with six cubes Copies a square	Dresses alone	Recognises three or four colours
5 years	Hops, stands on 1 foot or 10 sec	Copies triangle	Washes and dries face	Fluent speech

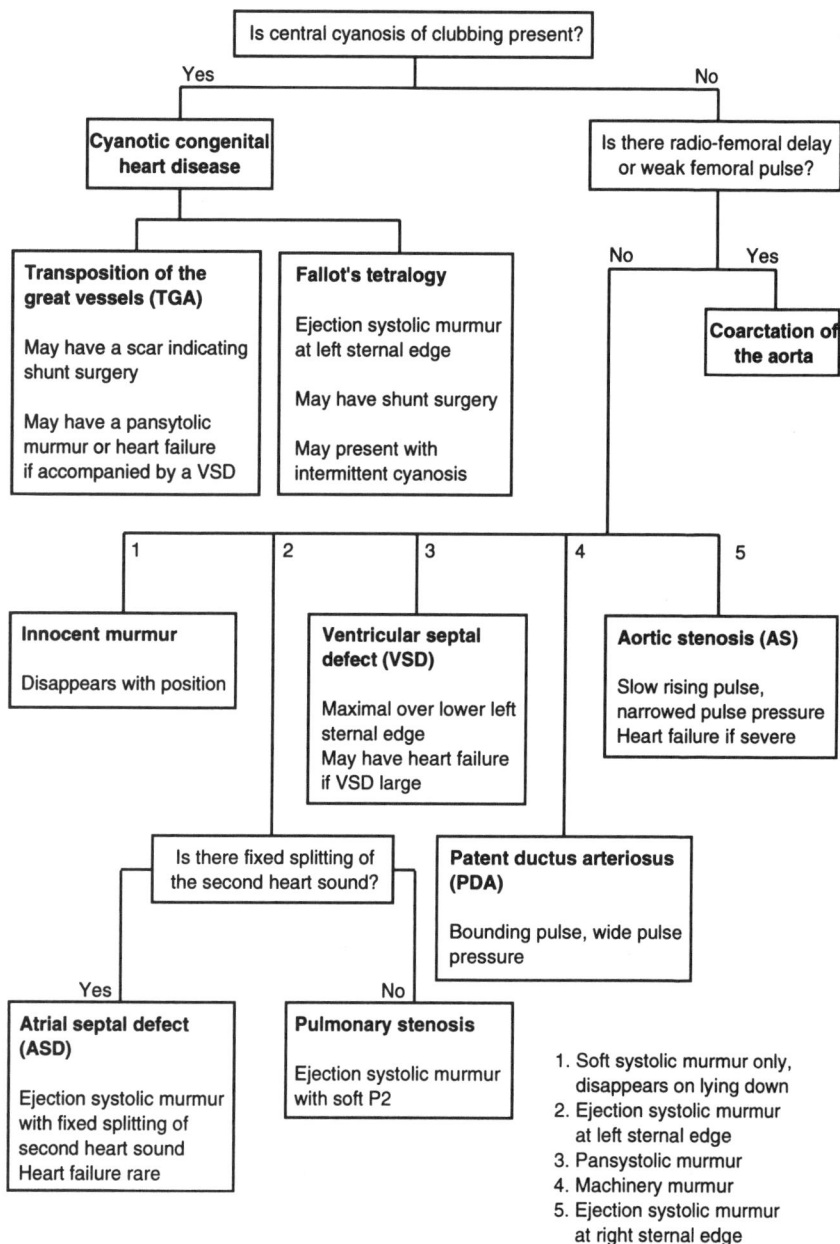

Figure 1   How to diagnose congenital heart disease.

(b) Inspection:

- Respiratory rate.
- Recession – subcostal and intercostal.
- Harrison's sulcus (indrawing of the lower ribs at the attachment of the diaphragm).
- Use of accessory muscles (especially sternomastoid).
- Chest deformities – e.g. pectus excavatum or pectus carinatum.
- Hyperinflation and increased antero-posterior diameter of the chest.
- Timing of the inspiration and expiration – increased inspiratory phase suggests stridor, increased expiratory time suggests lower airway obstruction.
- Audible stridor or wheeze without stethoscope.

(c) Percussion:

- Systematically percuss the front, back and both sides for dullness.
- Look for loss of cardiac dullness (sign of hyperexpansion).

(d) Auscultation:

- Is air entry equal on both sides of the chest?
- Listen for the presence of breath sounds, bronchial breathing, wheeze or stridor, and crepitations.
- Vocal resonance (listening while the child says '99'). This is sometimes useful in revealing areas of consolidation in older children.

Ask for peak flow readings.

Abdomen

The instruction to '*Examine the abdomen*' in a paediatric case may involve a range of conditions: a metabolic disorder, thalassaemia with hepatosplenomegaly; a surgical case with an inguinal hernia, liver disease, coeliac disease or renal problems.

Hence, in contrast to other systems, it is probably better to examine the abdomen first *before* deciding what general features to look for.

Examine older children on a bed with no more than one pillow. Younger or less cooperative children can be examined on their mothers' laps, and you may not be able to examine as comprehensively as described below. You must have warm hands before proceeding.

(a) Inspection:

- Previous scars.
- Distension.
- Peristalsis.

(b) Palpation:

- First ask the child if there is any pain.
- Watch the child's face while palpating.

- Expose the abdomen sufficiently (from xiphisternum to at least the inguinal regions).
- Perform *light palpation* in all four quadrants, noting any tenderness.
- Perform *deep palpation* for masses.
- *Palpate for the liver*, starting from below the umbilical region and gradually moving upwards with each inspiration. You should aim to feel for the edge of the liver on inspiration. The liver edge is often just palpable in children.
- *Palpate for the spleen* with the right hand, starting in the right iliac fossa and gradually moving towards the left hypochondrium. If the spleen is not palpable, place the child in a right lateral position with left hip and knee flexed, then palpate for spleen again.
- *Palpate for the kidneys.*
- *Check for hernias*, umbilical, para-umbilical, inguinal.
- *External genitalia.* Mention you would like to examine the external genitalia. The examiners will indicate whether this is necessary.

(c) Percussion:

- Over suprapubic region if an enlarged bladder is suspected.
- To assess the size of the liver or spleen.
- To elicit the cause for abdominal distension.
- To detect ascites.

(d) Auscultation:

- Generally necessary only if obstruction is suspected.

(e) General features:

What features to look for depends entirely on the findings of your examination of the abdomen and the hints given to you by the examiners. The following lists are examples; they are not exhaustive.

- Hepatosplenomegaly:
  — look for lymph nodes, anaemia, bruises (for leukaemia), and
  — look for stigmata of liver disease (clubbing, spider naevi, liver palms, jaundice etc.)
- Enlarged kidney – ask for blood pressure.

Neurology

Generally speaking, observation of the child is much more important than formal neurological examination of the tone, power and reflex.

Cerebral palsy (especially hemiplegic type), hydrocephalus (with or without spina bifida), and Duchenne muscular dystrophy are common cases in examination.

(a) General:

- Skin lesions (e.g. depigmented macules in tuberous sclerosis).

- Surgical scars (e.g. ventriculoperitoneal shunt for hydrocephalus).
- Head circumference.
- Talipes in spina bifida.
- Contractures in cerebral palsy.
- A protection helmet may indicate that the child has epilepsy.

(b) Observation:

For a young infant, stand back and observe for the following:

- *General posture* – poor head control may mean hypotonia, abnormal fisting, flexed elbow and plantar flexion on one side may mean hypertonia.
- Scissoring of the legs may mean spastic diplegia.
- *Persistent primitive reflexes* – e.g. asymmetrical tonic neck reflex.
- Observe which limbs appear to move most.
- Then proceed to examine tone and reflexes.
- Mention you would perform a developmental assessment.

For an older child stand back and observe the following:

- General posture – hemiparesis is often associated with closure of the hand and a flexed elbow on the affected side.
- Gait – e.g. characteristic hemiplegic gait with 'winging' of the affected arm while walking. Examine the sole of the shoe for the pattern of wear and tear.
- Ask the child to run or walk on tiptoe or walk toe-to-heel. The 'winging' of the affected arm may be more obvious in hemiplegia.
- Test for hand, foot and eye preference.
- (If Duchenne muscular dystrophy is suspected) ask the child to sit down on the floor and get up. He may need to 'climb with his hands up his legs' (Gower's sign).
- Proceed with an examination of tone, power and reflexes.
- Suggest developmental assessment.

Common syndromes seen in examination

(a) Physical signs of Down's syndrome:

General:

- Hypotonia.
- Short stature.
- Developmental delay.

Head and face:

- Delayed closure of the anterior fontanelle.
- May be a third fontanelle.
- Upward sloping palpebral fissures.
- Brushfield spots (white dots like a clock face in the iris).
- Epicanthic folds.

- May be a squint.
- Small mouth.

Hands and feet:
- Incurving fifth finger (clinodactyly).
- Single palmar crease.
- Wide gap between first and second toes.

Cardiovascular system:
- Increased incidence of atrioventricular canal defect, patent ductus arteriosus.
- VSD and Fallot's tetralogy.

Gastrointestinal:
- Increased rate of duodenal atresia and Hirschsprung's disease.

(b) Physical signs of Turner's syndrome:

- Short stature.
- Webbed short neck.
- Low hairline.
- Puffy feet and hands (in the newborn).
- Widely spaced nipples.
- 15 per cent have coarctation of the aorta.
- Lack of secondary sexual characteristics (in older untreated cases).

(c) Physical signs of neurofibromatosis:

- Skin nodules (neurofibromas).
- Café-au-lait spots.
- Axillary freckling.
- Acoustic neuromas (in some types of neurofibromatosis).
- May be scoliosis.
- May be increased blood pressure from renal artery stenosis or phaeochromocytoma.

(d) Tuberous sclerosis:

History:
- May have epilepsy.
- May have mental retardation.

Examination:
- Depigmented patches – 'ashleaf' depigmentation.
- Papules on face – adenoma sebaceum – in teenagers.
- Fibromata under nails.

TEST 1
Answers to Short Note and Case Commentary Questions

1 How would you assess a 3-month old baby whose head circumference lies below the 3rd centile?

Assessment

- Plot head circumference at birth – assess whether there is change in centiles.
- Plot the length, weight and head circumference of the baby. Does the small head simply reflect a small baby?
- Measure head circumference of parents.
- Palpate cranial sutures and fontanelles – early closure may indicate craniosynostosis.
- Look for abnormal head shape.
- Developmental assessment.
- Look for dysmorphic features.
- Consider investigations – skull X-ray for calcification; chromosomes; TORCH screen; urine for CMV.

2 A mother suspects that her 3-year old daughter has a squint. How would you assess the child? How would you advise the mother?

Assessment

- Decide whether it is a squint or a pseudo-squint:
  — examine for epicanthic folds and facial asymmetry,
  — examine whether the corneal light reflexes of the two eyes are symmetrical,
  — ocular movement,
  — cover test, and
  — alternate cover test.
- Assess visual acuity (by STYCAR letter test).
- Fundoscopy to exclude intraocular lesion (e.g. retinoblastoma).

Advice

- Refer the child to an orthoptist or ophthalmologist if any doubts whatsoever.
- Refractive errors are the most likely causes for squints. Appropriate glasses may be needed.
- If there is true squint, the child should be kept under observation by the orthoptist to prevent amblyopia.
- Established amblyopia may be treated by patching.

3 A 10-year old girl presents with secondary enuresis. Discuss the differential diagnosis. What questions would you ask her parents and how would you manage the child?

Differential diagnosis

No organic cause:
• Stress in the family.
• Stress at school.
• Recent bereavement.

Organic cause:
• Urinary tract infection.
• Diabetes mellitus.
• Diabetes insipidus.
• Neuropathic bladder.
• (If Afro-Caribbean), sickle-cell disease.

Questions to ask parents

• Duration of enuresis.
• Whether it is nocturnal, daytime or both.
• Whether it occurs at both weekends and weekdays.
• Family history of enuresis.
• Recent change in school.
• Recent stress in family, recent bereavement.
• Sibling rivalry.
• Fluid intake habit especially in the evening.
• The child's reaction to enuresis.

Management

• Reassure parents – 5% of 10 years old have enuresis; ultimate prognosis is good if organic cause is excluded.
• Exclude organic cause – midstream urine culture; urinalysis and urine specific gravity.
• General advice on fluid intake in the evening.
• Try star charts.
• Consider enuretic alarm method if above measures are ineffective.

4 A urine culture in a 6-month old boy showed more than 100 000 *E. coli* per mm^3. How would you manage the child?

• Ensure that the result was not due to contamination by repeating the urine culture.
• Give trimethoprim and then if necessary change according to sensitivity.
• Ultrasound scan of renal tract.

* Perform micturating cystourethrogram to exclude vesico-ureteric reflux.
* DMSA scan to look for scarring.
* Give prophylactic antibiotics until investigations are complete. Continue if vesico-ureteric reflux is present.

5 Write short notes on the consent to treat children under 16 years of age.

* Generally, the consent of a person with parental responsibility of the child must be obtained before treatment.
* This is usually the child's parents, but may be his or her guardian, adopted parents or local authority in certain situations.
* A child made a ward of court needs consent from the court.
* Under common law, one may proceed with emergency life-saving treatment if the persons with parental responsibility cannot be promptly located.
* If the child refuses to let the doctor contact his or her parents (e.g. prescription of contraceptive pills for girls), the doctor should:
  — persuade the child to discuss the proposed treatment with his or her parents or let the doctor discuss it with them,
  — if unsuccessful, the doctor should assess whether the child is competent to understand the treatment and its consequences (i.e. whether he or she is Gillick-competent),
  — if so, the doctor can treat the child if in his view it is in the child's best interests.
* Consent from the High Court must be obtained for all non-therapeutic treatments (e.g. sterilisation).

6 Briefly discuss the importance of childhood road-traffic accidents. List the measures which may reduce the incidence of childhood road traffic accidents.

Childhood road traffic accidents

* Account for about one quarter of all deaths of children under the age of 15.
* More than 300 children under the age of 15 die as a result of road traffic accidents each year.
* A pedestrian road-traffic accident is the single most common cause of accidental death in the 5–14 age group.
* The 'Health of the Nation' target aims to reduce the death rate for accidents among children aged under 15 by at least 33% by the year 2005. A reduction in road traffic accidents would be necessary to achieve this target.

Measures which may reduce the incidence of childhood road-traffic accidents

(a) Education:

* Education for the parents of the dangers through the media.

- Education of the children of the dangers.
- Increased public awareness
- Advertising (e.g. 'Kill your speed' campaign etc.).

(b) Legislation:

- Seat-belt regulations for children.
- Speed limits.
- Ramps in selected areas.
- Special measures near new schools.

(c) Improved design:

- Improved car design.
- Improved road design.

7   List the clinical features of atopic eczema in a 4-year old child. What treatments are available?

Clinical features

- Generalised dryness, thickening and lichenification of the skin.
- Itchiness.
- Excoriation.
- Found especially on the flexor surfaces of the limbs.
- Superimposed infection common.

Treatment

- Avoid irritants – use cotton rather than wool.
- Avoid soap – use soap substitutes.
- Use emollients and bath oils.
- Topical steroids – care taken for use on face.
- Oral antibiotics if complicated by bacterial infection.
- Consider dietary avoidance (if appropriate).

8   A 7-year old boy with known grand mal epilepsy presents in the Accident and Emergency Department with status epilepticus. Discuss your strategy in his management.

Management of the child

- Check the airway, breathing and circulation.
- Monitor pulse, breathing and blood pressure during the following treatment.
- Give facial oxygen.
- Insert intravenous cannula: take blood for investigations (glucose, urea and electrolytes, calcium, full blood count); give diazepam 0.2 – 0.3 mg/kg slowly.

- Give IV dextrose if the glucose level is low.
- If no response after a few minutes, give a second dose of diazepam.
- If no response, give IM paraldehyde.
- If no response, give IV phenytoin.
- If no response, consider IV clonazepam or chlormethiazole.
- If no response, the child may need general anaesthesia and ventilation.

9 **You have diagnosed diabetic ketoacidosis in a 10-year old with known insulin-dependent diabetes. Outline your immediate management of the child.**

Immediate management

- Initial rehydration of the child with intravenous normal saline or plasma (20 ml/kg).
- Replace intravenous fluid over 24 hours.
- Check glucose, urine and electrolyte and plasma osmolality, full blood count and arterial blood gas results.
- Consider potassium supplementation according to plasma potassium when the child starts to pass urine.
- Switch to dextrose/saline when blood glucose decreases.
- Examine for localised signs of infection, perform infection screen. Treat with antibiotics if signs of infection are found.
- Give short-acting insulin by continuous infusion pump, adjust rate according to response of BM.
- Give bicarbonate only if acidosis is very severe.

10 **Discuss the indications for circumcision (excluding cultural and traditional reasons). What complications may occur?**

It is important to distinguish between the normal non-retractile foreskin present in most boys during the first two years (at birth, less than 5% of boys have retractile foreskin; at 3 years of age the foreskin is retractile in 90% of boys) and true phimosis. The former ('physiological phimosis') is not an indication while true phimosis (skin at the end of the foreskin is tight and fibrotic) is an indication. Recurrent paraphimosis and balanitis if recurrent or associated with urinary tract infection are indicators.

Complications

- Haemorrhage occurs in 6–10% of circumcised neonates and is dangerous if a bleeding disorder is present.
- Post-operative infection.
- Meatal ulceration and stenosis – due to ammoniacal dermatitis (if still in nappies).
- Urethral strictures and fistulae.

- Injury to the glans.
- Inadequate excision of foreskin can lead to stricture.
- Excess removal of foreskin.
- Vessel thrombosis and gangrene.
- Anaesthetic complications (low incidence).

Circumcision is contraindicated in the presence of hypospadias or epispadias.

Case Commentaries

Case 1

1   The most important causes of acute lower respiratory illness are acute bronchiolitis, wheezy bronchitis and pneumonia. There is no clinical evidence to suggest a cardiac disorder. John has no bronchospasm and is not the usual age for acute bronchiolitis. The physical signs, pyrexia and listlessness suggest pneumonia. The previous chest infection, chronic cough and failure to thrive may be related to heavy maternal smoking, and social problems but one should consider an underlying disorder such as cystic fibrosis or immunodeficiency.

    As he is obviously quite unwell, admission to hospital is indicated as opposed to treatment with oral antibiotics at home. Initial management should include intravenous antibiotics to cover the most likely bacterial pathogens – *pneumococcus, haemophilus* and *staphylococcus*, maintaining hydration, oxygen saturation monitoring. Oxygen may be necessary and respiratory support may be necessary if the child deteriorates.

2   Recurrent respiratory infection, failure to thrive, abnormal stools and early finger clubbing suggest cystic fibrosis as the most likely underlying disorder. A sweat test is the single most important investigation. A sweat chloride level over 70 mmol/L on at least 100 mg sweat on two occasions confirms the diagnosis. A third confirmatory sweat test is often carried out at a later date. Pancreatic insufficiency is suggested by low faecal chymotrypsin levels.

3(a)   Following the diagnosis of a serious condition such as cystic fibrosis which has lifelong implications as far as treatment is concerned, it is important to discuss the different aspects of management on several occasions. The initial discussion should focus on management of the chest, nutrition and the management of pancreatic insufficiency. The nature of the condition should be discussed clearly and simply at the first meeting. At subsequent meetings, points raised at the first meeting should be reinforced and further information on possible long-term complications and genetic aspects should be discussed. It would be important to discover how much involvement the father has with John – he may need to be involved in aspects of the management of John's cystic fibrosis (e.g. chest physiotherapy).

    In discussing chest management, the following points should be raised:

    (i)   The importance of daily physiotherapy. John's mother should see the physiotherapist as soon as the diagnosis is established.

(ii) Physical exercise should be encouraged. When John is older, participating in sport is likely to be beneficial.

(iii) Reducing unnecessary contact with people having colds and acute respiratory infections.

(iv) His mother should be strongly encouraged to stop smoking.

(v) Antibiotics – long-term prophylaxis with flucloxacillin is useful (although some would disagree). A second antibiotic such as amoxycillin is added when John develops upper respiratory infections or if he develops a cough.

(vi) The importance of early treatment of chest infections should be emphasised.

The importance of a diet which is high in calories and protein should be emphasised. Fat intake should not be restricted. Children with cystic fibrosis require up to 50% more calories than unaffected children. Fat-soluble vitamins should be prescribed and if John's weight gain is not satisfactory, calorie supplements may be necessary.

The use of pancreatic enzyme supplements should be discussed and the following points made:

(i) The dose is gradually increased until stools become normal.

(ii) The dose is increased to cover foods which are more fatty.

(iii) Pancreatic enzymes are given with meals and snacks. Practical details of how to take the particular preparation are discussed.

(iv) Diarrhoea and a sore bottom may be due to too much pancreatic enzyme.

When discussing the prognosis with John's mother, one should point out that the outlook is very much better with modern treatment than in the past, and will continue to improve with advances in treatment. Currently, with proper treatment up to 80% of children survive into their late teens and about 50% survive to the age of 30.

The importance of regular follow-up should be emphasised.

The hereditary aspects should be discussed. One should ask about the possibility of John's parents getting together again and planning another child as this would obviously have genetic implications. Sweat tests should be carried out on John's sister.

Contact with the Cystic Fibrosis Research Trust should be offered.

3(b) Professionals involved with John's long-term management include the paediatrician, physiotherapist, dietician, social worker and general practitioner. Microbiologists are often useful when discussing antibiotic treatment for organisms cultured in sputum. Children with cystic fibrosis should be seen in special Cystic Fibrosis Clinics, and not in General Paediatric Clinics. At the clinics, the child is seen by the relevant specialists often including a cystic fibrosis nurse specialist.

3(c) The role of the general practitioner includes the following.

   (i) Reinforcement of the importance of regular physiotherapy, avoidance of contact with cigarette smoke and the points made in hospital discussions with John's mother.

   (ii) Ensuring that John is fully immunised, including immunisation against influenza.

   (iii) Early provision of antibiotics to cover upper respiratory infections and change in respiratory symptoms (e.g. onset of a cough).

   (iv) Liaison with the paediatrician should problems arise.

   (v) Providing support and encouragement to John's mother.

Case 2

1 Childhood obesity is rarely associated with underlying pathological conditions. However, most children with so called 'simple obesity' are tall for their age. Susan's height lies on the 25th centile which means that pathological causes should be considered, although simple obesity is still likely. Rare causes of obesity include hypothyroidism, Cushing's syndrome, hypopituitarism, hypothalamic tumours and congenital disorders such as Laurence–Moon–Biedl and Prader–Willi syndromes. Drug treatment (e.g. corticosteroids, sodium valproate) can cause obesity, but this is very unlikely in Susan's case as she has no significant past medical history.

Other useful information includes the following.

(a) Previous heights and weights – has Susan's growth fallen off in recent years? Is her obesity of recent origin?

(b) Heights and weights of parents and siblings. Is Susan's height appropriate for mid-parental height?

(c) Academic progress. Some pathological causes of obesity are associated with learning difficulties. Also in Susan's case, she may have been under-achieving because of her unhappiness due to obesity and perhaps parental divorce.

(d) Detailed diet history.

(e) How does Susan spend her leisure time? Does she spend it lying in front of the television? How much exercise does she take?

(f) Questions about the family dynamics. Was Susan upset by her parents' divorce? Does she see her father?

(g) Family history of cardiovascular disease, hypertension, diabetes.

The physical signs to look for include:

(a) Blood pressure.

(b) Presence of striae.

(c) Signs of hypothyroidism – these are not prominent in hypothyroid children.

(d) Signs suggesting a syndrome, e.g. polydactyly in Laurence–Moon–Biedl syndrome, phenotypic appearance of Prader–Willi syndrome.

(e) CNS examination including fundoscopy and visual field assessment.
(f) Evidence of puberty.
(g) Skin fold thickness measurements.

2 *Investigations.* If Susan's height is appropriate for her mid-parental height and if previous height measurements have not shown a fall-off in growth, the investigations required should be minimal but might include thyroid function tests (serum thyroxine and TSH) to exclude hypothyroidism, morning and evening plasma cortisol levels to exclude Cushing syndrome and bone age (pathological causes are often associated with delayed bone age). If previous height measurements indicate a significant fall-off in growth, one may have to consider pituitary function tests and chromosome analysis (Turner's syndrome).

3 The management of obesity is difficult, and a sympathetic but firm approach is needed. The reasons why it is important to lose weight should be discussed. The involvement of a dietician is important. Dietary advice includes limitation of sugary drinks, biscuits, cakes, chocolate and extra snacks, and modification of the calorie content of main meals. Modification of the dietary habits of the whole family is often helpful. Susan's mother is also obese, and she should be encouraged to participate in dieting with Susan.

Modification of Susan's lifestyle may be helpful, e.g. spending less time watching TV, walking as opposed to going by car, regular times for meals with reasonable intervals between meals. Increased physical activity and participation in sport could be beneficial although one should recognise that obese children may be self-conscious and reluctant to participate in team sports. Susan and her mother should be seen regularly. Encouragement and psychological support may well be necessary. If there is either a reduction in weight or even if the weight remains static when the height increases, this should be regarded as progress and praised accordingly.

4 The most obvious contributing factor towards her school refusal problem appears to be teasing by other schoolchildren. However, one should enquire about bullying in school. Susan may be reluctant to disclose this at first, and discussion with teachers about this possibility may help. One should also ask her teachers about Susan's academic prognosis. She may be experiencing difficulties and this could be contributing to her unhappiness. Another contributing factor could be separation anxiety especially following the experience of her parents' divorce. Susan's school refusal is recent and immediate return to school with psychological support should be the aim. Again, discussion with teachers is important. Involvement of a child psychologist or child psychiatrist may be indicated and individual or family therapy may be offered.

TEST 2
Answers to Short Note and Case Commentary Questions

1 What are the risk factors for congenital dislocation of the hips? Briefly describe how you would screen for congenital dislocation of the hips in the neonatal period.

Risk factors

- Positive family history.
- Girls.
- Breech delivery.
- Left hip.
- Caucasians.

Screening for congenital dislocation of the hips

- Ortolani's and Barlow's test. Abduct the thighs with the examiner's middle finger of each hand pressing forward on the greater trochanter. A 'clunk' felt suggests that the hips are dislocated. Abduct the thighs with the examiner's thumbs pressing backwards. A 'clunk' felt represents a dislocatable hip.
- Ultrasound may be used to confirm dislocation.
- Ultrasound all babies with risk factors.

2 What are the criteria for a good screening test? Briefly describe a common screening test for two disorders which fulfil most of these criteria.

Criteria for a good screening test

- The disease is an important health problem.
- There is a presymptomatic period.
- The test is able to identify a high proportion of those with the disease (high sensitivity).
- The test correctly identifies a high proportion of those without the disease (high specificity).
- The test is simple, cheap, and acceptable to the patients.
- Treatment is available, effective and cost-beneficial.

Two common screening tests

Guthrie's test for phenylketonuria and blood spot test for congenital hypothyroidism. A sample of blood by heel prick is taken. The blood spots taken at the same time as that taken for Guthrie's test are used for testing congenital hypothyroidism, and in some health regions, for cystic fibrosis screening by immunoreactive trypsin level. Both phenylketonuria and hypothyroidism, if diagnosed early, can be effectively treated by dietary restriction and thyroxine respectively. Untreated, both have severe detrimental effects on intellectual development and growth.

3 A 7-year old boy with known asthma presents in the Accident and Emergency Department with an acute asthmatic attack. List the signs and symptoms which would indicate the severity of this attack. What is your strategy for treating him?

Signs and symptoms which would indicate the severity of the attack

- Whether the child can talk in sentences, phrases, or words.
- Presence of cyanosis.
- Presence of tachycardia.
- Pulsus paradoxus more than 25 mm Hg.
- High respiratory rate.
- Intercostal and subcostal recession; indrawing at the Harrison's sulcus.
- Air entry (*Note*. Silent chest may indicate extreme severity).
- Severe reduction in peak flow.

Strategy in the treatment

- Administer oxygen with nebulised beta agonist (e.g. salbutamol).
- If no effect, admit. Repeat nebuliser regularly thereafter.
- Administer oral prednisolone (2 mg/kg/day) or intravenous hydrocortisone.
- Consider intravenous aminophylline (ask about current oral theophylline).
- If there is a deterioration in spite of these measures, the child may need ventilation.

4 A 16-year old girl presents with short stature and primary amenorrhoea. List the main causes and summarise your management of this girl.

The main causes

- Constitutional delay in puberty.
- Turner syndrome and other chromosomal abnormalities, e.g. XXX.
- Hypopituitarism, e.g. craniopharyngioma, cranial irradiation.
- Systemic disorders, e.g. severe asthma, cystic fibrosis, chronic disease.

Management of this girl

- Assess the growth chart especially regarding recent growth velocity.
- Check if there is a family history of delayed puberty.
- Examine for signs of puberty (e.g. breast development, pubic and axillary hair).
- Examine genitalia for imperforate hymen.
- Perform a fundoscopy and visual field examination.
- Consider the bone age.
- Consider chromosomal analysis, pituitary function tests or neuroradiological investigations if appropriate.
- Consider pelvic ultrasound scan.

From the above, decide whether the delayed puberty is consonant and physiological.

• Treat the cause.
• Consider oestrogen and progesterone to create a cycle.

5 You have a 5-year old boy with mild cerebral diplegia. What problems might the child experience? List the professionals who may be involved in his care, and briefly list their roles.

Problems he might experience

• Spasticity – Gross motor problems, e.g. a delay or difficulty in walking, contractures.
• Fine motor developmental delay, e.g. difficulties in manipulation.
• A squint.
• Psychological problems at school.
• Mental retardation and learning difficulties (less likely for cerebral diplegia than other forms of cerebral palsy).
• Epilepsy (less likely for cerebral diplegia than other forms of cerebral palsy).

Professionals who may be involved

• Hospital paediatricians – general paediatric care, treatment of epilepsy.
• Community paediatricians – developmental monitoring.
• Paediatric surgeons – operation on contractures.
• Physiotherapist – exercises to prevent contractures.
• Occupational therapist – to improve fine motor development.
• Ophthalmologists and orthoptists – to monitor and treat squints.
• Educational psychologists and special needs teacher – to provide special needs education, child may need statementing.
• Speech therapist.

6 A 9-year old boy presents with 3 days' history of fleeting joint pain, petechial rash over the buttocks, and abdominal pain. What is the most likely diagnosis? What are the other features and complications of this disorder?

The most likely diagnosis
Henoch–Schönlein purpura.

Other features and complications

(a) Skin:

• Urticarial rash.
• Oedema.

(b) Joints:

• May progress to joint swelling and effusion.

(c) Gastrointestinal (other than abdominal pain):

- Occult blood in stool or melaena.
- Intussusception.
- Vomiting.
- Haematemesis.
- Infarction and perforation (rare).
- Unnecessary laparotomy.

(d) Renal:

- Haematuria (microscopic or macroscopic).
- Proteinuria.
- Nephrotic syndrome.
- Hypertension.
- Focal proliferative glomerulonephritis.
- Diffuse proliferative glomerulonephritis leading to renal failure.
- Chronic renal failure.

(e) Central nervous system (rare):

- Epileptic fits.
- Nerve palsy.
- Coma.

7 A 4-year old boy is brought to you with speech delay. What are the possible causes, and how would you assess him?

Possible causes

- Secondary to mental handicap.
- Secondary to deafness (conductive or neural deafness).
- Isolated speech developmental delay.
- Dysarthria due to mechanical problems (e.g. cleft palate).
- Neurological disorders (e.g. cerebellar disorder).
- Autism.

Assessment

- Previous speech and developmental milestones.
- Hearing – any parental concerns and past screening results; hearing tests (audiometry).
- Inspection of tympanic membranes and external ears.
- Developmental assessment in other areas – to determine whether part of mental retardation or isolated.
- Assess quality of speech – whether evidence of dysarthria, receptive dysphasia or expressive dysphasia.
- Inspection of palate.
- Observe behaviour and interaction with parents (to detect autism).

8 List the clinical features of tuberous sclerosis in a child. What investigations would support your diagnosis?

Clinical features

- Learning disability.
- Epilepsy, infantile spasms as infants.
- Depigmented macules.
- Subungual fibroma, shagreen patches, facial angiofibromatomas in an older child.
- Behavioural problems.
- Retinal phakoma on fundoscopy.

Investigations

- Wood's lamp examination of the child.
- Wood's lamp examination of the parents.
- Plain skull X-ray.
- CAT scan and MRI scan.
- Echocardiogram – rhabdomyomata in young child.
- Intravenous pyelography or ultrasound may show renal disease (e.g. polycystic kidneys, renal cysts, angiomyolipomas).

9 What are the clinical signs of a ventricular septal defect? How would you evaluate the size of the defect clinically in a 3-month old child? How would you manage the child?

Clinical signs

- Loud pansytolic murmur loudest at lower left sternal edge, radiating throughout precordium.

If the size of VSD is moderate or large:
- Displaced apex beat.
- Thrusting apex beat.
- Thrill at lower left sternal edge.

Signs indicating a large defect

- Presence of heart failure – tachypnoea, tachycardia, hepatomegaly.
- Mid-diastolic murmur at apex.
- Loud pulmonary component of second heart sound (suggesting pulmonary hypertension).

Management

- Advise antibiotic prophylaxis before surgery or dental treatment.
- If the defect is small, it may be reviewed regularly for spontaneous closure. One must monitor the murmur to prevent development of pulmonary hypertension.
- Diuretics and/or captopril if evidence of failure.
- If the defect is large, it should be closed surgically.

10 What are the features of bruising associated with non-accidental injury? What conditions might be confused with non-accidental bruising?

Features of bruising associated with non-accidental injury

- The number or character of the bruises is often inconsistent with the history provided.
- Bruising in an infant not yet walking.
- Multiple bruises (most falls cause a single bruise).
- Fingertip bruising.
- Bruises of different colours.
- Bruising of the ears.
- Non-accidental bruising often occurs on soft surfaces (e.g. cheeks, abdomen, buttocks, genitalia or on the back or dorsum of the hand), while accidental bruises occur on bony contact points (e.g. forehead and shins).
- Slap marks leave linear marks on the cheek.
- Outlining of the bruising may correspond with a particular object (e.g. a stick, loop or cord, slipper).
- There may be other features of abuse (e.g. a torn frenulum, retinal haemorrhages, fractures, or failure to thrive).

Conditions which might be confused with non-accidental bruising

- Mongolian blue spots and bleeding disorders may cause confusion (always check FBC and film, prothrombin time, APTT, and bleeding time).
- Facial petechiae, conjunctival haemorrhage may occur with prolonged coughing bouts (e.g. pertussis or choking).
- Occasionally, it is difficult to tell if bruising is due to a genuine accident or NAI. One has to give an open verdict.
- Some rare connective tissue disorders cause easy bruising (e.g. Ehlers–Danlos syndrome).

Case Commentaries

Case 1

1 Breath-holding attack is the likely diagnosis for the two recent episodes. Fred's mother should be reassured that although these episodes may appear frightening, they are completely harmless and that Fred does not have epilepsy. Investigations (e.g. EEG) and treatment are not indicated and the prognosis is excellent. His mother can be assured that the episodes will stop before the age of 5 years, and often within a year or so.

2 Management strategy
(a) *Avoid positive reinforcement of his tantrums*
- Fred must not be given what he demanded after a tantrum.
- After a tantrum, indifference on the part of his parents is a better response than anger or an argument; such attention may only reinforce his behaviour.

- His parents should not show anxiety when he has tantrums or after a breath-holding attack.
- Praise or rewards should be given when he responds to a situation by not having a tantrum.

(b) *Consistency*
- Parental response must be consistent at all times.
- Both parents must agree on their responses which should be the same for both parents.

(c) *Other factors*
- Are there any changes within the family which may have led to Fred feeling insecure? There may be other family issues which need to be resolved.
- Do the parents respond to situations with anger and aggressive feelings? If so, this might reinforce the child's responses. Sometimes, the parents themselves need to examine and learn to control their own responses.

3 Iron deficiency is the most likely cause of Fred's anaemia. As he is thriving and otherwise well, this is very likely to be dietary in origin. Other causes such as malabsorption or chronic blood loss are much less likely. Malabsorption (e.g. coeliac disease) in a 2-year old who is thriving and has no gastrointestinal symptoms is very unlikely as a cause of iron deficiency. Chronic blood loss which may be occult, would have to be considered if his diet was found to have an adequate source of iron.

Appropriate investigations would be full blood count with white cell count (including differential count), platelet count, MCV and MCHC indices, blood film to rule out abnormal white cells and signs of haemolysis, reticulocyte count and ferritin level. These investigations would confirm the diagnosis of iron deficiency (microcytic hypochromic anaemia with a low ferritin); and exclude causes of anaemia such as haemolysis (e.g. congenital spherocytosis), acute leukaemia and aplastic anaemia.

4 A detailed assessment of Fred's diet should be carried out – he may be drinking excessive amounts of cows' milk and eating no or very little iron-containing foods. His parents should be advised to reduce Fred's milk intake to no more than 1 pint per day and to give him iron-containing foods (e.g. green vegetables, meat, iron-fortified cereals). He should be treated with an oral iron preparation which should be continued for 2 months after his blood count has returned to normal.

Case 2

1 Jack is having infantile spasms, sometimes referred to as salaam seizures.

2 An EEG should be carried out as soon as possible. This should show hypsarrhythmia which consists of high-voltage multifocal spikes, spike and wave

discharges, chaotic slowing and asynchrony. If an initial EEG shows non-specific abnormality, a sleep EEG will often show the characteristic hypsarrhythmia.

3 Underlying causes include the following.
- Perinatal hypoxaemia-ischaemia.
- Intracranial haemorrhage.
- Prenatal infection – CMV, toxoplasmosis, rubella.
- Post-natal infection – meningitis.
- Dysgenesis (e.g. tuberous sclerosis, Aicardi syndrome, cortical dysplasias, holoprosencephaly, schizencephaly, Sturge–Weber syndrome, neurofibromatosis).
- Metabolic disorders (e.g. hypoglycaemia, phenylketonuria, non-ketotic hyperglycinaemia, Leigh's syndrome, pyridoxine dependency).

Between 70–75% of children are found to have a specific cause for seizures. No underlying cause is found in the remainder.

4 *Investigations*
- Cranial CT scan. If this is normal, a MRI scan should be performed. This may show evidence of cerebral dysgenesis if the CT scan is normal.
- Wood's light examination of the skin to look for depigmented macules.
- TORCH screen and examination of urine for CMV.
- Urine metabolic screen, including organic acids.

If Jack is found to have tuberous sclerosis, it is important to exclude this diagnosis in his parents. Parental examination includes CT scanning, renal ultrasound scan, fundus examination, and Wood's light inspection of the skin.

5 Until recently, corticosteroids were regarded as the treatment of choice especially for cryptogenic cases (no underlying cause). However, this is associated with a mortality of up to 5% and other significant side-effects. In addition, steroids have not been shown conclusively to improve the long-term outcome. Vigabatrin is now considered to be the initial drug of choice for infantile spasms, and should be used in Jack's case. Steroids (e.g. prednisolone) may be considered if he does not respond.

Long-term developmental follow-up will be necessary for Jack. A diagnosis of infantile spasms is very serious and can be devastating for the family who may well require a great deal of support.

6 Jack's long-term prognosis is likely to be poor. Mental retardation occurs in 90% of cases and is severe in about 70% of them. There may be accompanying behavioural problems. Sixty-five per cent of children develop other forms of epilepsy, especially the Lennox–Gastaut syndrome and complex partial seizures.

7 Advice regarding future children will depend on the identification of any underlying cause. For example, if Jack and one of his parents are found to have tuberous sclerosis, the risk of tuberous sclerosis for each subsequent child will be 50% (this disease is an autosomal dominant disorder). If a metabolic disorder is detected (not a common cause of infantile spasms), the risk for further children will be 25% as these conditions are usually autosomal recessive in their inheritance. If Jack's infantile spasms are idiopathic, the recurrence rate is likely to be very low, and probably comparable with the risk for the general population.

TEST 3
Answers to Short Note and Case Commentary Questions

1 What are the advantages of administering the MMR (measles, mumps and rubella) immunisation to the health of the population and the child receiving the vaccine? What are the possible side-effects ?

Advantages to the health of the population

* Reducing the number of susceptibles in the population, increasing the herd immunity to all three infections (measles, mumps and rubella), and hence reducing the risk of an epidemic.
* Reduces or eliminates the risk of infants born with congenital rubella syndrome, by ensuring that (1) all women are immune at child-bearing age and (2) the level of susceptibles in the population is reduced

Advantages to the child receiving the vaccine

* Protects the child against all three infections.
* Reduces the risk of complications associated with each infection:
  — Measles: subacute sclerosing panencephalitis, encephalitis;
  — Mumps: orchitis and sterility in male; nerve deafness; and
  — Rubella: (for girls) congenital rubella syndrome in fetus.

Possible side-effects

* Mild pyrexia.
* Mild rash.
* Cervical lymphadenopathy.
* Mild parotitis.
* Convulsion (though risk is much smaller than natural measles).
* Encephalitis (risk is much smaller than natural measles).
* Subacute sclerosing panencephalitis (risk is very much smaller than natural measles).

2 You are asked to see a 12-hour old neonate with jaundice. What are the likely causes and how would you investigate and manage the child?

Likely causes – These are nearly always due to haemolysis

* Rhesus incompatibility.
* ABO incompatibility.
* Congenital spherocytosis.
* Glucose-6-phosphate dehydrogenase deficiency.
* Sepsis and intrauterine infection.

Investigation

- Bilirubin level (conjugated and unconjugated).
- Haemoglobin level.
- Blood film.
- Maternal and baby's blood group, Coombs' test.
- Septic screen – blood culture, urine culture.
- TORCH screen, urine CMV.
- G6PD (if appropriate).

Management

- Phototherapy or exchange transfusion (depending on bilirubin level).
- Treat underlying conditions (e.g. sepsis).

3 List the possible causes of faecal soiling. How would you manage a 5-year old boy with recent onset of faecal soiling?

Possible causes

Physical:
- Constipation with overflow.

Emotional:
- Poor toilet training.
- Emotional stress (expression of either regression or aggression).

Management

- Exclude constipation with overflow by abdominal examination, rectal examination. Sometimes X-ray is useful.
- Use of stool softeners (e.g. lactulose), stimulants (e.g. Senokot).
- Encourage high fibre diet.
- If the cause is constipation, an enema is useful.
- Star charts.
- Individual or family therapy if appropriate.
- Consider referral to a child psychiatrist.
- Admission for toilet training is sometimes indicated.

4 A 4-year old boy presents with a recent onset of bruises. What is the differential diagnosis and how would you investigate the child?

Differential diagnosis:
- Idiopathic thrombocytopenic purpura.
- Acute leukaemia.
- Platelet function disorder.
- Other clotting disorders.
- Child abuse.
- Accidental.

Investigations

- Examination for anaemia, lymph nodes, liver and spleen.
- Full blood count including haemoglobin, white cell count and platelet count.
- Blood film.
- Clotting screen – prothrombin time, APTT, bleeding time.
- Platelet function if bleeding time is prolonged and platelet count normal.
- Bone marrow biopsy if leukaemia or aplastic anaemia is suspected.
- Child abuse – localised bruises of different ages with associated finger marks, pattern of objects, slap marks. A social investigation if child abuse suspected.

5　A 12-month old boy presents with a 2 week history of persistent pyrexia, cervical lymphadenopathy, mouth ulceration, and recent peeling of the palms. What is the most likely diagnosis? List the clinical features and possible complications and briefly describe how he should be managed.

Most likely diagnosis

- Kawasaki disease (mucocutaneous lymph node syndrome).

Clinical features

- Prolonged fever.
- Conjunctivitis.
- Oral mucosal lesions – swollen lips and tongue.
- Redness, swelling of the hands and feet, peeling of the palms (third week).
- Rash.
- Cervical lymphadenopathy.

Complications

- Cardiovascular – coronary artery aneurysms, other arterial aneurysms, pericarditis, myocarditis.
- Hepatitis or obstructive jaundice.

Management

- Refer to cardiologist – ECG, chest X-ray, echocardiogram.
- (Within 10 days) Intravenous immunoglobulin in the acute phase.
- Salicylates in acute phase and at low dose for 6 to 8 weeks.
- Continue salicylates with or without dipyridamole until cardiac lesions are resolved.
- Follow-up.

6 List the characteristic features of acute bacterial meningitis in a 9-month old boy. List the common organisms responsible and possible complications.

Characteristic features

- Generally unwell.

- Apathy.
- Refusal to feed, vomiting.
- Irritability and not settling.
- Convulsions.
- High-pitched cry.
- Probable fever.
- Tense bulging fontanelle.
- Purpuric rash (meningococcal meningitis).
- Neck stiffness and positive Kernig's sign is often absent.

Common organisms

- *Haemophilus influenzae.*
- *Neisseria meningitidis.*
- *Streptococcus pneumoniae.*

Complications

- Subdural collection of fluid.
- Hydrocephalus.
- Sensori-neural deafness.
- Epilepsy.
- Cerebral palsy.
- Cranial nerve palsy.
- Shock.
- Inappropriate ADH secretion.
- Increased intracranial pressure.

7 A 3-year old boy presents with a first febrile convulsion lasting 2 minutes. How would you assess and manage the child? What advice would you give to his parents?

Assessment of the child

- History – family history of febrile convulsion or epilepsy.
- General well-being.
- Whether febrile before the convulsion.
- Take temperature.
- Examine for signs of infection – throat, tympanic membranes, chest, and signs of meningism.

Management

- Paracetamol and oral fluids.
- Usually admission to hospital.
- Monitoring of temperature and pulse.
- Lumbar puncture only if clinically indicated.
- Antibiotic treatment only if localised signs of infection are found.

Advice to parents

- Reassurance that it is a common disorder (4% of all children).
- About a 1 in 3 chance of a recurrence.
- It is not proven that prevention of recurrence reduce the risk of subsequent epilepsy.
- To remove excess clothing, and give paracetamol at the onset of future pyrexia.
- Advice on placing the child in left lateral position during a convulsion.
- May consider keeping rectal diazepam at home if the seizure lasts longer than a few minutes.

8 You were unable to palpate the testes of a male newborn infant during the routine examination. What are the possible causes and how would you manage the child?

Causes

- Retractile testes.
- Undescended testes (especially in premature neonates).
- Ectopic testes.
- Testes atrophied during development.
- Masculinisation of female infant.

Management of the child

- Re-examine in a warm room.
- Exclude masculinisation of a female infant (measure blood pressure, look for increased pigmentation, biochemical tests and karyotype if necessary).
- Examine for associated inguinal hernias.
- Needs follow-up regularly to ensure that testes have descended.
- If not, may need orchidopexy at about 2–3 years of age.

9 What are the characteristic features of toddler diarrhoea? What advice regarding management and prognosis would you give to the child's parents?

Characteristic features

- Between the ages of 6 months and 5 years.
- Variable stool frequency.
- Symptoms are worse later on in the evening than in the morning.
- Passage of undigested food particles.
- Growth and weight gain are satisfactory.

Advice

- Reassurance that there is no serious underlying disorder.
- Avoid drinking large amounts of orange squash.

Prognosis

- Very good.
- The vast majority are self-limiting.
- A minority persist with functional bowel disorder.

10 What problems are encountered by children born with cleft lip and palate? What is the paediatrician's role in management of the condition?

Problems in the neonatal period:

- Parental distress and shock.
- Possible admission to special care baby unit.
- Difficulty with breast-feeding.
- Problems with bottle feeding.
- Increased incidence of other congenital malformations.

After the neonatal period

- Repeated hospital admissions for surgery (sometimes delayed because of infection).
- Post-operatively – occasional infection, atelectasis, pneumonia, recurrent otitis media, hearing loss.
- Orthodontic problems, malposition of teeth.
- Speech defects – nasal escape, hypernasality, incompetence of palatal and pharyngeal muscles, difficulties with plosive sounds such as 'p', 't', and 'k'.
- Increased incidence of developmental problems.
- Psychological problems, e.g. teasing, bullying at school, lack of self-esteem.

Role of the paediatrician in the neonatal period

- Parental discussion and counselling, including an outline of the problems and management.
- 'Before and after surgery' photographs.
- Feeding management – teats with larger holes, lambs' teats.
- Discussion with plastic surgeon.
- Early involvement of orthodontist.
- Checking for other congenital malformations and developmental problems.
- Early treatment of infection.
- Early detection of hearing loss.
- Coordination of other specialists – plastic surgeon, orthodontist, otolaryngologist, dentist, social worker, speech therapist, dietician, psychologist.
- Continuing parental guidance and support.

Case commentaries

Case 1

1 Sarah's short stature may be due to constitutional growth delay although her height, which is quite far below the 3rd centile, would certainly warrant exclusion of other diagnosis. Parental heights have not been given, so familial short stature is possible, although the heights of her brothers do not support this diagnosis. The other causes which must be considered are hypothyroidism, hypothalamic or pituitary disease, Turner's syndrome, coeliac disease and occult renal disease.

2 *Further information*
   (a) Parental heights.
   (b) Other previous heights and weights for Sarah.
   (c) Family history of pubertal delay.

Particular attention should be paid to the following on physical examination.

   (a) Evidence of hypothyroidism (obvious signs are rare in prepubertal child).
   (b) Evidence of Turner's syndrome – neck swelling, low hairline, cubitus valgus, broad chest, short 4th metacarpal, widely spaced nipples and cardiac abnormalities. However, short stature may be the only obvious feature in some girls with the syndrome.
   (c) Fundoscopy and visual field examination.

Investigations
   (a) Thyroid function tests – thyroxine and TSH levels.
   (b) Full blood count – coeliac disease may present insidiously at this age with anaemia and short stature.
   (c) Chromosome analysis.
   (d) Blood urea, electrolytes and creatinine, urinalysis.
   (e) Bone age.

The above investigations should be carried out before considering pituitary function tests.

3 To explain Turner's syndrome, it is initially necessary to simply explain what chromosomes are. One would then explain that Turner's syndrome results when one X chromosome is missing. One could explain that certain physical features (which may be absent in Sarah's case) and short stature are features of the syndrome. One would explain that the ovaries fail to develop and that 90% of girls with Turner's syndrome will therefore require help to go through puberty. This takes the form of hormone replacement. Oestrogen is given alone in a gradually increasing dose for about 1–2 years, and then cyclical hormones (oestrogen and progesterone) are given to initiate menstruation.

One would explain that although girls with Turner's syndrome are not deficient in human growth hormone production, their growth often responds to daily subcutaneous growth hormone injection. Sarah's parents and Sarah should be reassured that such hormone treatment is safe and that side-effects are very unlikely.

4 The other important issue to discuss with Sarah's parents and Sarah, when she is older, is infertility. Spontaneous pregnancy is very rare in Turner's syndrome. Sarah may need psychological support for her infertility in the future. The possibility of an ovum donation pregnancy should be mentioned, although discussion on this could wait until Sarah is of child-bearing age.

Case 2

1 The following factors may have contributed to Tom's sleeping problem.
   (a) Normal children may experience varying degrees of separation anxiety when put to bed. The transition from an active environment, with lots of attention being paid to the child, to a quiet solitary environment can seem frightening to many normal children.
   (b) Tom's feeling of insecurity may be increased due to his parents' irregular working hours.
   (c) Sibling rivalry following the birth of his younger sister may be a contributing factor.
   (d) Parental anxiety about Tom's sleeping may have an effect on Tom.
   (e) The absence of established sleep routines or rituals. Taking Tom downstairs within 5 minutes after he starts crying reinforces this behaviour.

2 Tom's parents should be reassured that his sleep problem is not due to underlying illness.
   A detailed history of what happens prior to bedtime and how his parents respond to Tom's behaviour is important. Keeping a sleep diary which records Tom's sleep disturbance and his parents' responses over a period of a week or two is very useful. This can be used to establish a baseline of the problems involved and to monitor progress.
   Tom's parents should be offered the following advice.
   (a) Establish a regular routine before bedtime, e.g. a snack, followed by a bath and a story. Over-stimulation should be avoided at this time.
   (b) Try to eliminate or reduce naps taken in the afternoon.
   (c) Try not to show anxiety over his sleep problem in front of Tom.
   (d) Devote a fixed time to spend with him during the day to reduce his insecurity and feelings of sibling rivalry.
   (e) Do not respond to his crying by bringing him downstairs. Advising his parents to let him cry may not work, but advising them to let him cry for increasing periods of time before giving in to settle him calmly and sympathetically may be more effective.

(f) Rewarding him for not waking his parents may be effective.

In general, medication is not very effective in the management of a sleep problem. Prescribing a sedative may be misinterpreted by the parents that the problem is physical. Occasionally, a sedative may be used for a short period in an effort to break habits but generally one should try to avoid medication.

3 Advice regarding Tom's dental caries include:
   (a) Reduce his intake of between-meal snacks and drinks containing sugar.
   (b) Effective cleaning and brushing his teeth at least twice each day. A 3-year old child is not very effective in cleaning his teeth, and his parents will have to assume responsibility.
   (c) If there is no fluoridation of drinking water in the area they live in, fluoride supplements will be needed.
   (d) Some medications contain large amounts of sugar. Taking a drink of water and brushing teeth after medication is important.
   (e) Tom's parent should be advised to consult a dentist regarding his caries and for advice on dental hygiene.

TEST 4
Answers to Short Note and Case Commentary Questions

1 Describe how you would assess failure to thrive in a 2-year-old child with known recurrent wheezing whose weight is below the 3rd centile.

History

- Birth weight and previous weights to determine whether failure to thrive is recent.
- History of chronic cough; nature of cough.
- Parental height and determine mid-parental height.
- Duration and severity of wheeze.
- Symptoms of asthma to determine whether it is under control.
- Diet history.
- Other symptoms – diarrhoea, pale stools, urinary symptoms etc.

Examination

- Plot height on centile chart.
- Evidence of wasting.
- General examination – clubbing, cardiovascular system, chest shape, respiratory rate, presence of recession, listen to chest.
- Abdomen for liver and spleen, and distension.

Investigation

- Nil necessary if weight gain satisfactory and has been low birth weight.
- Full blood count for evidence of anaemia or infection.
- Serum urea, electrolytes and creatinine for evidence of renal failure.
- Calcium, phosphate and alkaline phosphatase for evidence of rickets.
- Urine for culture (for UTI).
- Faecal chymotrypsin.
- Faecal ova, cysts and parasites.
- Chest X-ray.
- Sweat test.
- Consider admission to hospital for observation and monitor of feeding and weight gain if significant failure to thrive and non-organic cause suspected.

2 What are the causes of precocious puberty? How would you assess a 7-year old girl with onset of puberty?

Causes

- Constitutional – normal but early activation of hypothalamic–pituitary–gonadal axis.

- Organic lesions of hypothalamic–pituitary region e.g. tumours, injury, infections, hydrocephalus.
- Endocrine causes – Cushing's syndrome, hypothyroidism, adrenal tumours.
- Ovarian causes – granulosa cell tumour or cyst or other tumours.
- Child abuse – administration of sex steroid.
- McCune–Albright syndrome.
- Neurofibromatosis.

Assessment

- History of the sequence of pubertal events – breast development, pubic and axillary hair and menstruation. Decide whether sequence is consonant.
- Plot heights – current and previous.
- Assess any associated psychological or social problems.
- Family history of puberty disorder.
- Staging of pubertal development.
- Visual fields, careful CNS examination.
- Bone age.
- Pelvic ultrasound.
- T4 and TSH, adrenal function.
- If any doubt about neurological signs or symptoms, perform a cranial CT scan or MRI scan.

3 **List the advantages and disadvantages of breast-feeding compared with bottle feeding.**

Advantages

- Appropriate nutrients – less risk of hypernatraemia, appropriate calcium:phosphate ratio, appropriate protein etc.
- Reduced chance of infection, especially gastroenteritis.
- Reduced chance of atopic disease, e.g. wheezy bronchitis, eczema, cows' milk protein intolerance.
- Enhanced mother-infant bonding.
- Cheaper.
- No risk of making feed over- or under-concentrated.

Possible disadvantages

- Problems with cracked nipples or mastitis.
- Inconvenience for some women.
- Risk of adverse side-effects of a drug in breast milk from mother, e.g. lithium, cytotoxic drugs.
- Inadvisable if mother has HIV disease in the United Kingdom, but breast-feeding is safer in underdeveloped countries.
- Breast milk jaundice (though this is harmless).
- Sometimes underfeeding.
- Some women may have inadequate supply of milk.

4 A 10-year girl with a good academic record presents with 3 weeks history of refusing to go to school. What are the possible causes? How would you manage the child?

Possible causes

- The diagnosis is school refusal.
- Separation anxiety of the child.
- Anxiety or phobia, e.g. travelling to school, certain school routines, specific teachers or classmates.
- Bullying, fear of teacher.
- More severe psychological disorder e.g. depression (rare).

Management

- Interview with the family to find out the cause.
- If a phobia, cognitive-behavioural approach may be used.
- Firm plan for early return to school, psychological support to child and parents.
- Discussion with teachers.
- Family therapy if problem is not resolved.

5 Write short notes on the following:
   (a) Strawberry naevus
   (b) Café-au-lait spots

Strawberry naevus

- Also known as superficial haemangioma.
- Usually appears a few weeks after birth, initially as a pale area.
- Grows rapidly in the first few months.
- Then remains stationary.
- Usually disappears before 10 years of age.
- Complications include ulceration and secondary infection, bleeding.

Café-au-lait spots

- Dark brown spots on the skin.
- Normal people may have less than five spots of more than 1.5 cm in diameter.
- Five or more café-au-lait spots, more than 5 mm diameter in the prepubertal child and more than 15 mm diameter in the post-pubertal child occur in patients with neurofibromatosis.

6 What basic principles underpin the changes contained in the 1989 Children Act ?

Basic principles

- The child's welfare should be the court's paramount consideration in any decision relating to the child's upbringing or administration of the child's property.

- Any delay in determining questions relating to the upbringing of a child is likely to prejudice the welfare of the child.
- The court will not make any order unless it considers that making the order is better than not making the order at all.
- Introduction of the concept of 'parental responsibility' – which includes all rights, duties, powers, responsibilities and authority which by law a parent of a child has in relation to the child and his or her property.

7 **You are called to see a 9-month old child with gastroenteritis. What are the clinical features of dehydration? What questions would you ask the parents? Briefly describe how you would manage the child.**

Clinical features of dehydration in a 9-month old child

- Thirst.
- Dry mucous membrane.
- Poor peripheral circulation and loss of skin turgor.
- Sunken eyeballs.
- Sunken fontanelle.
- Restless.
- Tachycardia.
- Hypotension.
- Reduced urine output.

Questions to ask the parents

- Duration, frequency and quantity of diarrhoea or vomiting.
- Fluid intake.
- Estimation of urine output – How often is the nappy wet?
- Has the baby been alert or drowsy?

Management of the child

- Assess whether hospital admission is necessary from estimated degree of dehydration.
- If not, give advice on oral rehydration therapy.
- Review the next day.
- If dehydration is severe, admit the child followed by measurement of urea and electrolytes.
- If oral intake is unsatisfactory, or if there is vomiting or severe dehydration, the child will require intravenous rehydration.

8 **What are the common organisms causing chest infection in a 5-year old boy for the first time? How would you treat him?**

Common organisms

- Viruses – Influenza, parainfluenza, adenovirus.
- Bacterial – *Pneumococcus*, *Haemophilus influenzae*.
- *Mycoplasma pneumoniae*.

Treatment

• Antibiotics – amoxycillin, third-generation cephalosporin, will cover both *Pneumococcus* and *Haemophilus influenzae.*
• Erythromycin is the treatment for *Mycoplasma* infection.

9 **Severe haemophilia A has been diagnosed in a 1-month old boy whose grandfather, a haemophiliac, died from an intracranial haemorrhage 26 years ago. He is the first child of the couple. What points would you raise in discussions with his parents?**

• Discussion on the nature of the condition – hereditary deficiency of Factor VIII, blood does not clot adequately.
• Main problems likely to occur when he is ambulant – he may have spontaneous bleeding into joints and muscles, risk of bleeding after dental extractions, and surgery. (emphasise he will need good dental care).
• Bleeding from cuts is unlikely to be a major problem.
• Parents will be concerned about internal bleeding, especially intracranial haemorrhage – reassure the parents that this is rare.
• Discuss Factor VIII treatment – now more effective and safe products are available. Reassure the parents about HIV infection.
• Discuss regular supervision from haemophilia centre and rapid access to Factor VIII treatment.
• Advise that he will not need special schooling and should be treated as normal. Only contact sports should be avoided.
• Advise not to circumcise.
• Advise full immunisation (injections are given subcutaneously).
• Advise hepatitis B immunisation.
• Discuss genetic aspects – 50 % of their sons likely to have haemophilia, 50 % of daughters carriers.
• Give the address of Haemophilia Society.

10 **What is the definition of juvenile chronic arthritis? How would you classify the disorder?**

Definition
Chronic arthritis developing before the sixteenth birthday and persisting for more than 3 months with the exclusion of other diseases (infections, malignancy, connective tissue diseases, such as SLE and dermatomyositis, reactive arthritis, blood diseases, such as haemophilia, orthopaedic conditions such as Perthes' disease).

Classification

1 *Systemic onset disease*
e.g. fever, rash, anaemia, lymphadenopathy, hepatosplenomegaly.

2 *Polyarticular onset (five or more joints)*
  (a) Rheumatoid factor negative.
  (b) Rheumatoid factor positive (juvenile rheumatoid arthritis).

3 *Panciarticular disease (less than five joints)*
  (a) Antinuclear factor positive – usually young girls.
  (b) Antinuclear factor negative.
  (c) HLA B27 positive – usually older boys.

Case Commentaries

Case 1

1 *Other points to be elicited from the history*
  • Whether Jack had been in contact with the suspected case of meningitis.
  • Any recent infectious disease in the family.
  • Any history of epilepsy or other neurological disease in the family.
  • Whether Jack was on any regular medication.
  • What regular medication his father took and where the medication was kept.
  • Any history of a recent head injury.

Physical signs to look for

  • Respiratory rate – evidence of respiratory depression.
  • Heart rate and rhythm, blood pressure.
  • Peripheral perfusion and capillary refill time.
  • Presence of a purpuric rash suggesting meningococcal disease. If present, it is an indication for immediate parenteral benzylpenicillin.
  • Other neurological signs, particularly pupillary size, symmetry and reaction.
  • Fundoscopy – retinal haemorrhage or papilloedema.
  • Examination of head externally for bruises and swelling.
  • Signs of child abuse, e.g. bruising.
  • Work out a Glasgow Coma Scale (GCS) score.

2 *Differential diagnosis*
  • Meningitis.
  • Encephalitis.
  • Intracranial haemorrhage – subdural haematoma following head injury, spontaneous intracranial bleeding, e.g. bleeding from an AV malformation.
  • Drug ingestion – particularly sedatives in this case.
  • Other intracranial pathology, e.g. tumour or abscess – much less likely than the above.
  • Metabolic conditions including hypoglycaemia.

3 *Immediate management by the general practitioner*
  • Ensure the airway is clear, breathing is regular, and heart rate and BP are stable.
  • Ensure that he is placed in the left lateral (recovery) position.
  • Perform BM stix test to check for hypoglycaemia.
  • Arrange urgent admission to hospital.
  • Stay with the patient until the ambulance arrives.

4 The most likely explanation for Jack lapsing into coma and recovering spontaneously is that he has taken his father's medication, probably a benzodiazepine prescribed for his anxiety state. He had been unsupervised for a period during the afternoon.

5 His parents should be advised about keeping medication securely out of Jack's reach. One should also ask if his father's drugs were in a child-proof container. General advice on prevention of childhood accidents would also be useful during the discussion.

Case 2

1 *Assessment*
Further information from the history on:

- Whether there was any recent viral infection.
- Whether there was any recent drug ingestion.
- Family history of urinary infection, recent haematuria (for IgA nephropathy, benign familial haematuria), deafness (for Alport's syndrome), polycystic disease, renal stones, TB, renal failure, other renal disease or bleeding disorders.
- Whether an ultrasound scan was carried out in the antenatal period, and its results.
- Whether there was any recent trauma.

Investigations

- Repeated urine examination for blood and protein and microscopy and culture (to exclude urinary tract infection).
- Urine calcium to creatinine ratio (to exclude idiopathic hypercalcuria).
- Full blood count and film, blood urea, electrolytes, creatinine, plasma proteins and serum C2 level.
- Coagulation screen (although this is an uncommon presentation of a bleeding disorder), but a sickle screen should be carried out if the parents are Afro-Caribbean.
- Ultrasound examination of urinary tract to exclude major anatomical abnormalities, polycystic disease and tumour.
- If all the above investigations are normal, one may reassess the situation before proceeding to more invasive investigations such as intravenous pyelography, micturating cystourethrography or renal biopsy.

Of crucial importance at this stage is the determination of urine abnormalities during the hospital admission, particularly in relation to finding blood in the nappy. Genitalia and anus should be inspected after reported bleeding episodes.

2 The likely diagnosis is Münchhausen syndrome by proxy.

3 *Steps to be taken*
- At this stage it is important to show that the nappy blood does not belong to the child. This is best done by carrying out blood grouping and DNA analysis on blood specimens from the nappy, baby and mother. This may involve assistance from the regional forensic laboratory.
- Confront the mother with the information in a non-accusatory manner.
- It may be helpful to discuss the case with a psychiatrist first. Occasionally, it may be necessary for the psychiatrist to assess the mother in case there is a risk of self-harm.
- Information should be obtained from the GP, health visitor, nursery workers, and hospital notes about the mother's previous health. The case should also be discussed at this stage with the social services.
- It is important that the child should stay in hospital with the parents excluded for a week or so, to demonstrate that the symptom is absent when the child's parents are not present.
- If there is a risk of removal of the child, an Emergency Protection Order will be necessary.

4 *Further information*
- Information regarding mother's previous health (medical and psychiatric) may be useful (e.g. whether she has shown evidence of Münchhausen syndrome herself).
- Social services may be able to provide information (e.g. whether mother has been in care herself).
- Information on the extended family and their problems may be useful.
- Whether there is adequate support for the mother should the decision subsequently be taken to allow the child to go home.
- The relationship between the parents, especially as the father has been noted to be an aggressive individual.
- Whether the child's mother has fabricated the symptom to draw attention to her problems with a difficult cohabitee, or perhaps seek refuge in the hospital.

5 *Points to raise at a subsequent case conference*
- Clear factual account of the presenting symptoms, the child's stay in hospital, and the evidence for Münchhausen syndrome by proxy.
- The harmful effects of this syndrome - the fact that the child has already been subjected to venopunctures and hospital admission and could well have been subjected to more invasive, unpleasant investigations at the instigation of the mother.
- Other long-term effects of the syndrome, e.g. some children have eventually succumbed to enforced invalidism or Münchhausen syndrome themselves as a result of fictitious illness. Some children have even died.

6 *How can the family be helped?*

- Help and support will depend on the mother's acceptance or denial of what she has done.
- If there is complete denial and hostility of the parents, it will probably be necessary for the child to be removed while social services are continually assessing the family.
- Psychiatric evaluation will be necessary.
- If the mother accepts what has happened, supervision at home may be possible with support for the family. Detailed assessment of the mother's relationship with her child and her ability to care adequately for the child will be necessary.
- If a difficult and perhaps violent relationship with the child's father has been at least partly responsible for her mother's actions, separation of the couple may be appropriate.
- The general practitioner and health visitor should be kept fully informed. The GP should be aware that referral should be to one named paediatrician, who is fully aware of the situation. This one paediatrician can, if appropriate, initiate future referrals to other specialists. This avoids the risk of several specialists seeing the child without being aware of the overall picture.

Continuing communication with the general practitioner will be important. His role will be central in monitoring the medical and emotional well-being of the child and any future siblings. The general practitioner should be involved early and encouraged to attend case conferences.

TEST 5
Answers to Short Note
and Case Commentary Questions

1 **A systolic murmur was noted on routine examination of a 2-year old boy who otherwise appears healthy. List the clinical features which would suggest underlying congenital cardiac abnormality and the clinical features which would suggest that this is an innocent murmur.**

Clinical features suggesting underlying cardiac abnormality

- Presence of cyanosis.
- Presence of clubbing.
- Weak or delayed femoral pulses (suggests coarctation).
- Abnormal pulse volume.
- Abnormal cardiac impulse (heave).
- Abnormally loud or soft second heart sound.
- Fixed splitting of second heart sound (suggests atrial septal defect).
- Pansystolic murmur.
- Diastolic murmur.
- Murmur louder than 2/6.

Clinical features suggesting innocent murmur

- Relatively short systolic ejection murmur, no radiation, best heard lower left sternal edge.
- High pitched blowing short systolic murmur in pulmonary area Grade 1 or 2.
- Venous hum – anterior upper chest. Disappears by compressing jugular venous system.

2 **What are the risk factors for deafness in a child? Describe the routine screening test in infancy for deafness, and state when the test should be performed.**

Risk factors for deafness

- Positive family history.
- Neonatal unconjugated hyperbilirubinaemia.
- Maternal infection (e.g. rubella, cytomegalovirus, toxoplasmosis, syphilis).
- Drugs – aminoglycoside (e.g. gentamicin).
- Cerebral palsy.
- Previous meningitis.
- Frequent middle ear infections.
- Syndromes (e.g. Treacher Collins, neurofibromatosis).

Distraction test

- Three adults needed.
- Performed in quiet room.
- Child seated on mother's lap.
- The second adult sits about a 1m in front of the child, and distracts the child using, for example, an attractive toy.
- The toy is gradually withdrawn.
- The third adult produces a low-pitched sound of pre-determined volume at the level of the child's ear.
- A positive response occurs when the child locates the source of the sound by head turning.
- The test is repeated with high-pitched sound.
- To pass the test, a positive response of at least two out of three trials.

When the test should be performed

- Between 7–8 months.

3 List the clinical signs of Down's syndrome. What other conditions may be associated with Down's syndrome?

Clinical signs

(a) General:

- Hypotonia in infancy.

Head and neck:

- Characteristic head shape – brachycephaly and flat occiput.
- Delayed closure of anterior fontanelle.
- Possible third fontanelle.
- Redundant skin nape of neck.

(b) Face:

- Upward sloping of palpebral fissures.
- Epicanthic folds.
- Brushfield's spots (in periphery of iris).
- Possible cataracts.
- Small low set ears.
- Flat nasal bridge.
- Protruding tongue.

(c) Hands and feet:

- Short, broad hands.
- Clinodactyly 5th fingers.
- Single palmar crease.
- Distal axial triradius.
- Widened gap between first and second toes.

(d) Development:

• Mental retardation.

Other associated conditions

• Congenital heart disease – e.g. atrioventricular canal defect, ventricular septal defect, Fallot's tetralogy.
• Duodenal atresia.
• Acute lymphoblastic leukaemia.
• Leukaemoid reactions.
• Hypothyroidism.
• Diabetes.
• Atlantoaxial instability.
• Increased susceptibility to infections.
• Hearing loss.
• Obstructive sleep apnoea.
• Subsequent Alzheimer's dementia.

4   What are the characteristic clinical features of nephrotic syndrome? What investigations would confirm this diagnosis?

Clinical features

• More common in boys and between the ages of 2 and 5.
• Oedema initially periorbital.
• Oedema becoming generalised.
• Abdominal pain.
• Poor urine output.
• Pleural effusions.
• Ascites.

Investigations to confirm diagnosis

• Urinalysis shows gross proteinuria. Some children have haematuria.
• Serum albumin – hypoalbuminaemia.
• Cholesterol and triglyceride levels high.

5   A 6-week old male infant presents with projectile vomiting after every feed, but appears hungry afterwards. What is the most likely diagnosis? List the possible biochemical abnormalities. How would you confirm the diagnosis? What is the treatment?

The most likely diagnosis
Congenital hypertrophic pyloric stenosis.

Possible biochemical abnormalities

• High bicarbonate level and pH (alkalosis).
• Low chloride level.
• Hypokalaemia.

Confirm the diagnosis

- Test feed – palpation of pyloric tumour in the right hypochondrium.
- Ultrasound if diagnosis is uncertain.

6 A healthy 8-year old boy was found to have a random blood pressure measurement of 140/110. What are the possible causes? What investigations would you perform?

Possible causes

- Incorrect measurement or use of narrow blood pressure cuff.
- Renal causes – glomerulonephritis, polycystic disease, reflux nephropathy.
- Cardiovascular cause – coarctation of the aorta.
- Other vascular causes – renal artery stenosis.
- Endocrine – Cushing's syndrome, some types of congenital adrenal hyperplasia.
- Tumours – phaeochromocytoma, neuroblastoma.
- Drugs – steroids.
- Primary hypertension.

Investigations

- Repeat blood pressure measurement.
- Examination for radio–femoral delay.
- Urinalysis, urine specific gravity, urine culture.
- Urea and electrolytes, creatinine.
- Renal ultrasound, abdominal ultrasound.
- Other renal investigations if indicated.
- Urine catecholamines.
- Morning and evening cortisols.

7 A 7-year old child presents with a bald patch on his scalp. What are the possible causes? Briefly describe the treatment for each cause.

- Hair pulling (trichotillomania) – Find out any recent emotional upset and manage accordingly.
- Fungal infection (tinea) – oral griseofulvin.
- Partial alopecia areata – No effective treatment.

8 Discuss the presentation, management and diagnosis of intussusception.

Presentation

- Repeated screaming attacks accompanied by pallor and drawing up of legs.
- Baby often looks extremely unwell during attack, but is initially well between attacks.
- Followed by vomiting which becomes bile-stained.
- Passage of blood per rectum, classically 'redcurrant jelly'.
- Occasionally diarrhoea is present.

- Typical intussusception is palpable as a sausage-shaped mass in right hypochondrium (uncommon if ileo-ileal).
- Occasionally presentation may imitate acute neurological illness, with profound listlessness.

Diagnosis

- Plain X-ray often shows signs of obstruction and a soft tissue mass.
- Ultrasonography is often useful.
- Clinical features may be sufficient for diagnosis.

Management

- Adequate resuscitation, rehydration, and correction of electrolyte upset.
- Non-operative reduction with air or barium enema (also confirms diagnosis) – contraindicated if peritonitis or perforation are present, or patient is shocked.
- Operative reduction if contraindications are present or non-operative reduction has failed.
- Careful monitoring of patient after non-operative reduction.

9   What clinical features would make you suspect Duchenne muscular dystrophy in a 4-year old boy? What is his likely prognosis? What points are important in discussing management with his parents?

Symptoms

- Difficulty climbing stairs.
- May have delayed walking (most walk at the usual age).
- Waddling gait, frequent falls.
- Difficulty with running and jumping.
- Some may have developmental delay.

Signs

- Proximal muscle weakness, legs more than arms.
- Pseudohypertrophied calf muscles.
- Gower's sign on rising from the floor.
- Waddling gait.
- Lordotic posture.

Points in discussing management

- Importance of physiotherapy in preventing contractures.
- Avoidance of prolonged bedrest – can cause deterioration in muscle weakness.
- Avoidance of obesity.
- Discussion of special educational needs – may not be required until later.
- Some boys have learning difficulties which need assessment.
- Genetic aspects – discuss X-linked inheritance, carrier detection and prenatal diagnosis.
- Emphasis on the long-term availability of support.

10 List the problems which may be encountered during the first year of life by a baby born to a HIV positive mother. What advice would you give regarding immunisation?

- May be uninfected and asymptomatic – vertical transmission rate in Europe is 15–20%.
- May be infected, but asymptomatic.
- Non-specific presentation – failure to thrive, diarrhoea, lymphadenopathy, hepatomegaly, splenomegaly, fever, impaired growth.
- Recurrent bacterial infections, e.g. *Haemophilus, Pneuomococcus, Salmonella*.
- Opportunistic infections – candidiasis, *Pneumocystis carinii* pneumonia, CMV infection.
- Lymphoid interstitial pneumonitis – may be asymptomatic although cough and dyspnoea may gradually develop.
- HIV encephalopathy – developmental delay, loss of milestones, microcephaly, progressive motor signs with spasticity.
- Social problems, e.g. maternal illness or death, maternal drug abuse, parental guilt, financial problems, HIV 'stigma'.

Advice regarding immunisation

Children should receive all routine immunisations, including MMR, but excluding BCG. Should receive killed polio vaccine instead of oral live polio vaccine.

Case commentaries

Case 1

1 The most likely diagnosis is gastro-oesophageal reflux. This is common and often mild in babies who are otherwise well and thriving. One should ask about the exact amount of milk taken at each feed as over-feeding may encourage vomiting. One should also ask about the feeding technique and winding. Matthew may be bringing up feed with his wind. The main alternative diagnosis to consider at this age is pyloric stenosis, although this is less likely in a baby who is thriving. Cow's milk intolerance can cause vomiting, but this is unlikely in a baby who is thriving without other symptoms.

In assessing the situation, the following information is important.

- The amount of milk taken at each feed.
- Any difficulties with winding.
- The amount vomited (this may be over-estimated by parents).
- The character of the vomiting – is it projectile? Projectile vomiting is characteristic of pyloric stenosis although vomiting as a result of reflux can be forceful.
- The presence of blood in the vomit. This would suggest oesophagitis although blood in the vomit is not uncommon in pyloric stenosis.
- Other symptoms – respiratory symptoms, loose stools.

In addition to a full physical examination, a test feed for evidence of pyloric stenosis should be carried out. Palpation during a feed is carried out with the fingers of the left hand in the area just lateral to the right rectus and below the liver edge. The tumour which feels like an olive, comes and goes throughout the feed.

At this point, assuming that one's findings are negative, it is valid to assume that the baby has mild reflux. Reassure the parents and suggest thickening the feeds with Carobel.

2 Matthew's respiratory symptoms and the choking episode indicate the need for further investigations, which should include:

- A chest X-ray to look for evidence of aspiration.
- Barium swallow. This may show the presence of a hiatus hernia and/or oesophageal reflux. However, significant reflux may be missed during a barium swallow examination.
- Twenty-four hour oesophageal pH monitoring. This is the best method for detecting significant reflux and should be undertaken if reflux is suspected despite an unhelpful barium swallow.
- Isotope scan to detect reflux and aspiration. This is occasionally carried out but has a low sensitivity for detecting abnormality and is not regarded as routine.
- Full blood count to detect anaemia due to reflux oesophagitis. If present, faecal occult blood tests are indicated. If significant oesophagitis is thought likely, endoscopy should be considered to evaluate its severity.

3 *Management strategy.* The long-term outlook is good with symptoms abating before the age of 2 years in at least 60% of children. Medical treatment is therefore initially indicated and surgery in the form of fundoplication only indicated if complications such as choking and aspiration do not promptly respond to medical treatment. Serious complications such as recurrent apnoea and significant haematemesis would lead to earlier consideration of surgery.

Medical treatment
- Sleeping in the prone position with the top of the mattress raised.
- Feed thickening (e.g. with Carobel).
- Cisapride. This prokinetic drug increases the resting tone of the lower oesophageal sphincter and stimulates gastric emptying.
- If oesophagitis is thought to be present, an H_2 receptor blocker such as ranitidine is indicated.

Case 2

1 Specific questions regarding the pain.

- *Character* – whether it interferes with everyday activities.

- *Time relation to events* – whether it was related to a specific event (e.g. brother leaving home, mother returning to work).
- *Time relation to school* – whether it occurs at weekends or on holiday; whether it is worse on Sunday nights or Monday mornings.
- *Time relation to food* – whether it is related to meal times or types of food; whether it causes night waking.
- *Associated symptoms* – nausea, vomiting, pallor, headache, bowel symptoms, urinary symptoms.

2 Further information.

- *Previous height and weight measurements* – may be obtained from school health service.
- *Problems at school* – academic performance, fear or dislike of a particular teacher, bullying.
- *Father's illness* – whether gastrointestinal symptoms were significant components of his illness; Louise's reaction at the time of his death.
- *Mother's health* – whether she is anxious, tense and conscientious, whether she finds it difficult to cope, whether her job is stressful, her mother's age at menarche.
- *Family history* – recurrent abdominal pain, dyspepsia, peptic ulcer, bowel disease, urinary tract, migraine.
- *Brother's health and relationship with Louise*
- *Louise's other symptoms to suggest anxiety*, e.g. sleep disorder, undue fears.

3 Investigations.

- Urinalysis and urine culture.
- Full blood count and ESR – elevated ESR might indicate organic disease.
- Blood electrolytes, creatinine.
- Liver function tests.
- Thyroid function tests.
- Chromosome analysis.

The justification for these tests is the combination of short stature, abdominal pain and poor appetite. Previous height measurements might suggest that her growth velocity over the years has been reasonable, but this information often takes a few weeks to obtain.

Further investigations

- *Bone age* – if very delayed, may point to organic disease (e.g. hypothyroidism, coeliac disease).
- *Helicobacter* antibodies – consider doing this test if a family history of peptic ulcer emerges. Otherwise, the result may cause confusion.

- Coeliac antibodies – consider if full blood count shows anaemia or bone age is very delayed.
- Abdominal ultrasound scan – although this is likely to be normal, the test is non-invasive. A normal result can provide strong reassurance, especially if Louise and her mother are worried about cancer.

4 Future management.

At this point, it is important to avoid further, possibly more invasive investigations which may give the message that organic disease is likely to be present and cause further anxiety. Strong reassurance is likely to be helpful, emphasising that the examination and all the tests have been normal. There may have been a particular, perhaps unspoken, fear of cancer in view of her father's illness and death. At the same time, one should emphasise that although organic disease is absent, the pain experienced is very real and can be severe. A discussion of the nature of recurrent abdominal pain is helpful, mentioning that it can affect 10–15% of children and comparing it to headaches which some adults experience. Its relationship to anxiety should be discussed.

One should then address any source of anxiety. Concern about school work, bullying or fear of one particular teacher will necessitate liaison with the school. One needs to be aware of any maternal anxiety present, and the mother may need support if she finds it difficult to cope following the death of her husband or if she finds her job stressful. Referral to an adult psychiatrist may be necessary. It may be necessary to explore her relationship with Louise.

Louise's height, together with absence of signs of puberty, may be other sources of anxiety, and should be discussed. Her height is likely to be related to parental height and her absence of pubertal change to constitutional delay. An estimation of her likely final height should be given in addition to reassurance about pubertal change.

Continuing follow-up is important to keep a check on symptoms, growth and pubertal development. It might be necessary to consider further investigation if there are no pubertal changes in a year or so. Should abdominal pain continue in the face of normal growth, weight gain and examination, referral to a child and adolescent psychiatrist should be considered.

TEST 1
Answers to Multiple-Choice Questions

1 **A** = False **B** = True **C** = True **D** = False **E** = False

The Court Report on Child Health Services ('Fit for the Future') was published in 1976. On the whole, it recommended a multidisciplinary approach to child health services and public health aspects of paediatrics. It recommended a multidisciplinary team in each health district for the treatment of handicapped children, and at least one trained community consultant paediatrician per health district. These two recommendations have been mostly implemented. It also recommended that the child health visitor should be involved with preventive as well as curative aspects of child health.

2 **A** = False, **B** = False **C** = False **D** = False **E** = False

The education of children with special needs has changed from a medical perspective, in which education is tailored according to the child's medical diagnosis and prognosis, to an educational perspective, in which education is tailored to the child's individual educational needs. The cause of the disability, the IQ of the child, the prognosis and medical treatments given are not important questions to ask from the educational perspectives. Instead, the individual educational strengths and weaknesses are assessed, the skills the child has already acquired, the range of skills the child must acquire are determined, and a plan for teaching is made. Instead of deciding which type of school the child goes to on the basis of the IQ, the decision is now based on the child's needs and the resources available in different schools. Instead of having different curricula for different children, the same curriculum (the National Curriculum) is provided for all children. However, the methods, rate, and level of delivery are different according to the child's ability.

3 **A** = False **B** = False **C** = True **D** = False **E** = False

Sex education in schools is one of the most controversial issues in education. At present, the school governors have a statutory requirement to decide whether or not sex education features in the school curriculum. Their decision usually considers parents' views, children's home background, culture and religion, the school's mission, and resources available. If they decide in favour of sex education, they must make a written policy regarding the content and organisation of sex education delivery. All teachers can be involved in sex education.

4 **A** = False **B** = False **C** = True **D** = True **E** = False

Factors associated with successful foster placements include younger age of children at placement, a short period of being in care; the presence of children of similar age group in the placement family; realistic expectations of parents and foster parents. The most important factor is probably the child's enthusiasm to be placed in foster care.

5   **A** = False   **B** = False   **C** = True   **D** = True   **E** = True

Stillbirth rate is the number of babies born dead with a gestational age of at least 24 weeks per 1000 *total* births.

Perinatal mortality rate is the number of stillbirths and deaths in the first 7 days of life per 1000 *total* births.

Infant mortality rate is the number of infants dying in the first 12 months of life per 1000 live births.

Neonatal mortality rate is the number of babies dying in the first 28 days of life per 1000 live births.

Post-neonatal mortality rate is the number of babies who die between 28 days and 1 year of age per 1000 live births.

6   **A** = False   **B** = True   **C** = True   **D** = True   **E** = False

Child Health Clinics play an important part in child health surveillance. They are staffed by health visitors, community paediatricians and receptionists. Immunisations, health education, developmental and growth assessments, counselling and management of specific problems can be carried out. However, some parents may not find the clinics easily accessible, and hence home visiting is still necessary.

7   **A** = False   **B** = True   **C** = True   **D** = True   **E** = False

Many advantages of parent-held records have been demonstrated. Communication between health professionals and parents is enhanced and parents are more involved. There is increased availability of records when the child is seen, and parents seldom lose the record. They are generally well-liked by both parents and health professionals.

8   **A** = True   **B** = True   **C** = True   **D** = True   **E** = True

Oral polio vaccine is a mixture of live virus of strain types 1, 2 and 3. It must be given three times to ensure that immunity develops against all three strains of polio virus. It produces both local gut and systemic immunity, and is excreted in faeces. It is contraindicated in pregnancy and in those with immunodeficiency.

9   **A** = True   **B** = False   **C** = True   **D** = False   **E** = True

Pertussis vaccine is a killed vaccine against different serotypes of the organism. It is usually given as a combined vaccine with tetanus and diphtheria. It should not be given to those who have had a severe reaction to a previous dose, or to those with progressive neurological disorder. It is particularly important that those with chronic illness such as cystic fibrosis receive the vaccine.

10   **A** = False   **B** = False   **C** = True   **D** = False   **E** = True

Generally speaking, skimmed milk should not be given to children under the age of 3 years, as it does not contain sufficient calories for the growing child. Sugary food should be avoided because it encourages dental caries. Highly salty food should be avoided in children.

11 **A** = False   **B** = True   **C** = True   **D** = True   **E** = True

Growth hormone deficiency may cause hypoglycaemia and a small penis in the newborn period. It may be associated with other endocrine deficiencies as in panhypopituitarism. Affected children are short with delayed bone age. They may be obese with a facial appearance which seems young for their age.   *R*   *SC human GH replacement*

12 **A** = True   **B** = False   **C** = True   **D** = True   **E** = True

An average 9-month old child can sit unsupported for more than 10 minutes but cannot walk around furniture until about 1 year of age. He or she can transfer objects from hand to hand at the age of 6 months, and approach objects with the index finger at 9 months.

13 **A** = False   **B** = True   **C** = False   **D** = True   **E** = False

The presence of a torn frenulum strongly suggests child abuse by pushing a feeding bottle hard inside the mouth. A generalised purpuric rash suggests reduced numbers of platelets (e.g. idiopathic thrombocytopenic purpura), or meningococcal septicaemia. The presence of retinal haemorrhages suggests injury due to shaking. Toddlers occasionally sustain forehead bruising after falls and most normal 8-year old boys have bruised shins.

14 **A** = False   **B** = False   **C** = False   **D** = True   **E** = False

Tympanometry measures the sound reflected back from the tympanic membrane when the middle ear pressure is varied, and it helps detect middle ear disease such as serous otitis media. It is therefore not a hearing test. It can be performed on a child of any age, as it requires little cooperation from the child. A normal result shows maximum compliance when the middle ear pressure is 0 mmHg. A flat curve indicates lack of compliance of the tympanic membrane, and may indicate fluid in the middle ear.

15 **A** = True   **B** = True   **C** = False   **D** = True   **E** = True

In non-accidental injury, the parents either tend to be over-protective or show a lack of interest and concern for their children. They may delay seeking medical advice and treatment without good cause. Their account of the injuries often changes with questioning. Localised bruising, especially of different ages, is typical of non-accidental injury. Generalised bruising may be due to thrombocytopenia or deficiencies in clotting factors. Torn frenulum may result from forced feeding, and is typical of non-accidental injury, but may occasionally occur due to genuine accident. A 9-month old baby is not ambulant, and fracture of the tibia is strongly suggestive of non-accidental injury.

16 **A** = True   **B** = True   **C** = False   **D** = True   **E** = False

Fever of more than 5 days duration and at least four out of five of the following features are necessary to diagnose Kawasaki's disease: non-purulent conjunctivitis; changes in the oral mucous membranes; changes in the extremities (erythema, oedema, peeling in the second or third week); rash (usually macular); and cervical lymphanopathy. ESR, C reactive protein and platelets are usually elevated. The most serious complications are coronary artery aneurysms, and a follow-up echocardiogram should be performed. Early treatment with aspirin and intravenous immunoglobulin is indicated.

17 **A** = False   **B** = True   **C** = False   **D** = True   **E** = False

A wheal of less than 5 mm is regarded as negative, while a wheal of more than 1 cm is regarded as positive. A wheal of between 5 mm to 1 cm is borderline, and other clinical details must be taken into account. A wheal of more than 1.5 cm indicates sensitivity to tuberculin, and is strongly suggestive of active tuberculosis, especially if there is no previous history of BCG immunisation. Although the Heaf test is the most reliable of the multiple puncture tests, the Mantoux test is more reliable than the Heaf test.

18 **A** = True   **B** = True   **C** = False   **D** = True   **E** = False

Babies who are small for their gestational age babies have reduced glycogen reserve in the liver. They also have a higher surface area to body weight ratio, and are hence prone to hypothermia. They may have polycythaemia due to a high erythropoietin level. As congenital abnormality is often associated with low birth weight, a higher proportion of babies who are small for their gestational age have congenital abnormalities. Respiratory distress syndrome is more likely to occur in preterm babies.

19 **A** = True   **B** = True   **C** = False   **D** = False   **E** = True

The distinction between unconjugated and conjugated hyperbilirubinaemia is important. Severe unconjugated hyperbilirubinaemia may cause kernicterus, but not conjugated hyperbilirubinaemia. Conjugated hyperbilirubinaemia indicates cholestasis, and can be due to neonatal hepatitis, biliary atresia, metabolic disease such as alpha-1-antitrypsin deficiency, sepsis or congenital infection. Ultrasound of liver and gall bladder, HIDA scan and liver biopsy should be considered if extrahepatic cholestasis is suspected.

20 **A** = False   **B** = True   **C** = False   **D** = False   **E** = True

Leavell classified prevention into primary, secondary and tertiary. Primary prevention seeks to prevent the onset of a disease. Secondary prevention seeks to detect a disease at a pre-symptomatic stage. Most screening programmes are examples of secondary prevention. Tertiary prevention seeks to minimise the damage of disease after symptoms appear. Hence addition of fluoride to drinking water to prevent dental caries, preconceptual genetic counselling and immunisation are examples of primary prevention. Neonatal screening for hypothyroidism and amniocentesis to detect congenital abnormalities are examples of secondary prevention.

21 A = True   **B** = False   **C** = False   **D** = True   **E** = False

An average 2-year old can go up stairs one foot per step, and downstairs two feet per step, holding on. (It is more difficult to go downstairs than upstairs.) He or she can build a tower of six or seven cubes, and imitate a vertical stroke with pencil and paper, but the child cannot give full name or copy a circle with pencil until he or she is 3 years of age.

22 A = False   **B** = True   **C** = False   **D** = True   **E** = True

Coeliac disease is caused by the effect of the alpha-gliadin component of gluten on small intestinal mucosa. The proximal small bowel is mainly affected. The majority of children present between 9 months and 2 years of age. The disease may cause mixed microcytic and macrocytic anaemia due to iron and folate deficiency. All children suspected of coeliac disease should have a jejunal biopsy performed. Subtotal villous atrophy and crypt hypertrophy are characteristic.

23 A = True   **B** = True   **C** = True   **D** = True   **E** = True

Most children with chronic constipation have no organic pathology. However, Hirschsprung's disease should be considered if constipation has been present from early infancy. Poor fibre and fluid intake, anal tears and anal fissures are common predisposing factors. A laxative and stool softener may be used together, and a simple behavioural programme such as the use of star charts may be effective.

24 A = True   **B** = True   **C** = True   **D** = True   **E** = True

Pneumonia can be caused by a large number of organisms in the immuno-compromised. The illness is often severe and life-threatening. Viruses include cytomegalovirus, chickenpox, herpes simplex and measles. *Pneumocystis* is a protozoan organism which can cause pneumonia in the immunocompromised especially children with AIDS. Prophylaxis with cotrimoxazole reduces the incidence. Fungal infection such as *Candida* can also cause pneumonia in the immunocompromised.

25 A = False   **B** = True   **C** = False   **D** = True   **E** = False

Sodium cromoglycate is effective in asthma prophylaxis only if given by inhalation. It is free from any significant side-effects, and is recommended as a first-line prophylactic drug. It can be given regularly to prevent an attack, but is ineffective once an attack has started. It is usually given four times daily.

26 A = True   **B** = True   **C** = True   **D** = True   **E** = True

Inhaled salbutamol immediately before exercise is often effective in preventing an exercise-induced attack for up to 2 hours. Both sodium cromoglycate and inhaled steroids are effective in preventing seasonal asthma. Nocturnal asthma often indicates that the disease is poorly controlled. Peak flow measurement is a good objective method of monitoring the disease, especially for older children. Children aged 7 or older should be able to perform peak flow reasonably well.

27 **A** = True   **B** = False   **C** = False   **D** = True   **E** = False

Acute epiglottitis usually affects children aged 2 to 6 years. It is caused by *Haemophilus influenzae* Type B (HIB) in the majority of the cases. The child becomes acutely unwell with high pyrexia and toxicity, subcostal recession, hoarseness and inability to speak, drooling of saliva, dypsnoea and stridor with upper respiratory tract obstruction. The clinician must not examine the throat, as this may convert a partial airway obstruction to a complete airway obstruction. If this condition is suspected, the consultant anaesthetist, paediatrician and ENT surgeon should be summoned urgently for a diagnostic laryngoscopy, and intubation if the diagnosis is confirmed. A lateral neck X-ray is unnecessary, and may put the child in further distress and cause complete obstruction. Fortunately, this disease is now rare following the introduction of HIB vaccine.

28 **A** = True   **B** = False   **C** = False   **D** = True   **E** = True

The cardinal signs of heart failure in infants are tachycardia and tachypnoea followed by hepatomegaly. The absence or reduction of femoral pulses may indicate coarctation of the aorta. Raised jugular venous pressure and ankle oedema are good indicators of heart failure in adults, but not in infants.

29 **A** = False   **B** = True   **C** = False   **D** = False   **E** = True

Innocent murmurs are either Grade 1 or 2 in intensity and short and systolic. They are commonly heard along the left lower sternal edge where they are medium pitched, vibratory or musical and vary with position of the child. Hyper-extension of the back and neck will usually lead to their disappearance. Innocent pulmonary murmurs are brief, high pitched and best heard in the second left parasternal space. The venous hum heard in the neck or anterior upper chest is due to turbulence in the neck veins. This is a continuous humming sound and can be increased or made to disappear by altering head position. Apart from the venous hum, innocent murmurs are never pansystolic or diastolic. There should be no other abnormal cardiovascular findings such as thrills or abnor-malities of the heart sounds.

30 **A** = True   **B** = True   **C** = True   **D** = True   **E** = True

Congenital heart disease is caused by genetic and environmental factors. Some chromosome abnormalities are associated with a higher risk of congenital heart disease. For example, Down's syndrome has a high incidence of congenital heart disease, especially ventricular septal defect and atrioventricular septal defect. Turner's syndrome is associated with coarctation of the aorta. Those with a positive family history are also more at risk. Maternal illness (such as diabetes), infection (such as rubella) and exposure to drugs and alcohol (as in foetal alcohol syndrome) are associated with a higher incidence of congenital heart disease.

31 A = True   **B** = True   **C** = True   **D** = True   **E** = False

Renal disease, such as chronic glomerulonephritis, neophropathy due to vesico-ureteric reflux, and Wilms' tumour, is the commonest cause of secondary hypertension. The most important vascular cause is coarctation of the aorta. Endocrine causes include Cushing's disease, hyperaldosteronism, and salt-retaining types of congenital adrenal hyperplasia. Rarely, phaeochromocytoma and neuroblastoma can cause sustained or paroxysmal hypertension.

32 A = False   **B** = True   **C** = True   **D** = False   **E** = False

About one-third of children who have a first febrile convulsion will have a recurrence. This is more likely if the first convulsion occurs before the child's first birthday, if it is prolonged, or if there is a positive family history. The duration of a recurrence is often shorter than the first seizure. Parents should be advised to give paracetamol during subsequent febrile illnesses. Long-term anticonvulsant treatment is rarely indicated for children with recurrent febrile convulsions, although some parents whose children may be at risk of prolonged seizures are given a supply of rectal diazepam for home use.

33 A = False   **B** = True   **C** = True   **D** = True   **E** = True

Migraine occurs in about 5% of schoolchildren. It is more common with increasing age, but the incidence decreases after puberty in boys. Hence, it is more common in boys than girls before puberty, but it is more common in girls after puberty. There is very often a positive family history. Food (especially chocolate and cheese), stress, fatigue, hormones (e.g. puberty in girls and oestrogen in contraceptive pills) may all precipitate attacks of migraine.

34 A = True   **B** = False   **C** = False   **D** = False   **E** = True

Hemiplegic cerebral palsy may result from an intrauterine thromboembolic event and neuroimaging (CT or MRI scan) may show evidence of previous infarction. About one-third of patients have seizures but a minority (approximately 25%) have learning difficulties. The arm is often more affected than the leg. In severe cases, the arm is flexed and adducted and the hand closed. The affected leg may be shorter.

35 A = False   **B** = True   **C** = True   **D** = True   **E** = False

Tuberous sclerosis is a neuro-ectodermal disorder with an autosomal dominant inheritance. Skin abnormalities include ash-leaf depigmentation in infancy, which is clearly seen with Wood's light, shagreen patch, periungual fibroma, and adenoma sebaceum (facial angiofibromata). However, adenoma sebaceum usually develops after puberty. Neurological manifestations include epilepsy and mental retardation. A CT scan may show multiple nodules projecting into the ventricles, forming the appearance of 'candle gutterings'. They are often calcified and can be seen on a plain skull X-ray.

36 **A** = False   **B** = False   **C** = True   **D** = False   **E** = True

Haemophilia A, is a sex-linked recessive disorder, and results from Factor VIII deficiency. Factor VIII is an important component in the intrinsic clotting system. Hence, prothrombin time (which measures the extrinsic pathway) is normal, but the APTT is prolonged. Children with haemophilia should never be prescribed aspirin or given intramuscular injections. DDAVP (desmopressin) is useful to cover minor surgical procedures in mild cases, but is ineffective in severe haemophilia.

37 **A** = True   **B** = True   **C** = True   **D** = False   **E** = False

Acute glomerulonephritis is usually post-infectious (e.g. following streptococcal infection), and may present with non-specific symptoms such as lethargy, anorexia, and abdominal pain. Specific symptoms and signs include hypertension, haematuria, smoky brown urine, oedema and oliguria.

38 **A** = False   **B** = True   **C** = False   **D** = True   **E** = False

Growth hormone deficiency may be congenital or acquired. Acquired causes include craniopharyngioma and cranial irradiation. Temporary partial growth hormone deficiency occurs in some physical conditions as well as psychosocial deprivation. Growth hormone deficiency is not an all-or-nothing phenomenon, but ranges from mild to total deficiency. As growth hormone is released in pulses and has a short half-life, a random growth hormone level is unhelpful. Growth hormone production is assessed using a HGH stimulation test – clonidine, glucagon and insulin-induced hypoglycaemia. (Caution is necessary with the last test.) The treatment of growth hormone deficiency is once daily subcutaneous injection of growth hormone.

39 **A** = True   **B** = False   **C** = False   **D** = True   **E** = False

A child with diabetic ketoacidosis is usually severely ill and may present with vomiting, dehydration, and abdominal pain. The first priority should be rehydration with isotonic sodium chloride (i.e. 0.9% normal saline) after restoration of extracellular fluid volume in the first few hours. Total fluid deficiency should be corrected over 48 hours. A short-acting insulin infusion should be given via a syringe pump, and adjusted according to the blood glucose response. Four per cent dextrose should be added to the IV fluids when the blood glucose falls to around 10 mmol / L. Cerebral oedema is the main cause for death associated with diabetic ketoacidosis, which is why total fluid replacement is carried out gradually over 48 hours.

40 **A** = True   **B** = False   **C** = False   **D** = True   **E** = True

Signs of severe dehydration include high fever, depressed fontanelle, dry mucosa, sunken eyes, reduced skin turgor, poor peripheral circulation, drowsiness, and oliguria (or anuria).

41 A = True   **B** = False   **C** = True   **D** = False   **E** = True

Scabies is caused by the mite *Sarcoptes scabiei* which burrows into the skin and lays eggs. These hatch into larvae, which travel to the surface and form burrows. The burrows are usually on the hands and wrists, especially in the interdigital webs. The patient complains of intense itching and an extensive rash. It is transmitted by close contact, not by clothing. The whole family should be treated irrespective of symptoms. Untreated scabies may be complicated by bacterial infection.

42 A = True   **B** = True   **C** = False   **D** = False   **E** = True

For a murmur to be innocent, there must be no other cardiovascular signs or symptoms. The most common innocent murmur is heard along the left lower sternal edge and varies with position. Hyperextension of the neck and back often causes it to disappear. Innocent pulmonary murmurs also occur. These are brief blowing early systolic murmurs no more than Grade 2 in intensity. The third type of innocent murmur is the venous hum, which is heard over the upper chest in systole and diastole. This is caused by turbulence in the jugular venous system and is diminished or made to disappear by gentle pressure over the neck veins.

43 A = True   **B** = False   **C** = False   **D** = False   **E** = False

Infants with pyloric stenosis lose acid in their vomitus, resulting in hypochloraemic alkalosis. They have a high bicarbonate level and a low chloride level. The pH is high, and glucose level is usually normal. Potassium levels are often deceptively normal but hypokalaemia may become apparent when rehydration and correction of the metabolic alkalosis is in progress. However, nowadays many babies present quite early when biochemical changes are minimal.

✳ **44 A** = True   **B** = False   **C** = True   **D** = True   **E** = True

Older children with coeliac disease may present insidiously with short stature or pubertal delay and not have a history of intestinal symptoms. Although antibody measurement can be useful in screening, a small intestinal biopsy is necessary for diagnosis. Treatment with a gluten-free diet involves exclusion of wheat, rye, barley and oats. If untreated, there is a risk of developing lymphoma in adult life.

45 A = False   **B** = True   **C** = True   **D** = True   **E** = True

In Europe, the vertical transmission rate from mother to baby is 15–20%. The rate is increased if the mother has symptomatic disease and/or a low T4 cell count. AZT during pregnancy may reduce the transmission rate.

46 A = False   **B** = True   **C** = True   **D** = False   **E** = False

Lymphoid interstitial pneumonitis, the more frequent occurrence of bacterial infections, and the rarity of Kaposi sarcoma are features of paediatric not adult HIV infection. Lymphoid interstitial pneumonitis is slowly progressive and the child may be asymptomatic for many years, whereas pneumocystiis infection has a high mortality and a high incidence of neurological disease in survivors. Children with HIV infection should be immunised normally with the exception of BCG. Killed polio is used rather than live polio vaccines.

47 A = False **B** = True **C** = True **D** = True **E** = True

Intussusception occurs mainly in children aged 5 to 9 months with two-thirds of the cases occurring in boys. About 85% of cases are ileo-colic. The classical presentation is with repeated screaming attacks accompanied by pallor and followed by vomiting and rectal bleeding ('redcurrant jelly'). A few infants present with marked listlessness and apathy suggesting an encephalopathic illness. Abdominal ultrasound examination may be useful in making the diagnosis.

48 A = False **B** = True **C** = True **D** = False **E** = True

A prolonged bleeding time occurs in thrombocytopenia or in conditions where platelet function is abnormal, for example, following aspirin ingestion. In Von Willebrand's disease, platelets are unable to adhere to damaged endothelium. A prolonged bleeding time also occurs in congenital disorders of platelet function such as Glanzmann's disease.

49 A = False **B** = False **C** = False **D** = False **E** = True

Precocious puberty is much more common in girls where it is also more likely to be constitutional. The appearance of early puberty in a boy should prompt a search for a cause, particularly an intracranial neoplasm. Although growth initially accelerates with advanced bone age, one of the main concerns in precocious puberty is the reduced final height due to earlier epiphyseal fusion.

50 A = True **B** = True **C** = False **D** = True **E** = True

Abnormalities associated with Wilms tumour include aniridia, hemihypertrophy, other genitourinary abnormalities and the Beckwith–Wiedemann syndrome. Gastro-oesophageal reflux can cause wheezing either via reflexes originating in the lower oesophagus or via aspiration.

In addition, asthma, through changes in intrathoracic pressure can predispose to gastro-oesophageal reflux. Tuberous sclerosis is associated with depigmented macules, adenoma sebaceum (angiofibromata) and shagreen patches. The incidence of café-au-lait patches characteristic of neurofibromatosis is not increased in tuberous sclerosis.

51 A = False **B** = False **C** = False **D** = True **E** = True

Pyloric stenosis is more common in boys and is absent at birth as recent ultrasound studies have shown. The vomiting is projectile and not bile stained although haematemesis can occur. The association with gastro-oesphageal reflux has been referred to as the Rovaralta syndrome and may cause persistent vomiting after pyloromyotomy.

52 A = False   **B** = True   **C** = False   **D** = True   **E** = False

The majority of children with infantile spasms have an onset between 4 and 9 months. A specific aetiology may be found in most cases. Common causes include cerebral dysgenesis or malformations (e.g. tuberous sclerosis), preceding hypoxic-ischaemic insult, preceding intracranial haemorrhage (e.g. intraventicular haemorrhage), intrauterine infection, neonatal meningitis and metabolic conditions. Mental retardation is a sequel in 80 – 90% of cases. Although corticosteroids can control the spasms, they do not alter the long term outlook and have a significant incidence of side-effects. This has led some paediatricians to prefer vigabatrin to which infantile spasms may show a good response.

53 A = True   **B** = True   **C** = False   **D** = True   **E** = True

Hypoglycaemia is the most common complication occurring in infants of diabetic mothers but the incidence of hypocalcaemia, hyperbilirubinaemia, polycythaemia, and respiratory distress syndrome is also increased. Renal vein thrombosis may be related to hyperviscosity and coagulation abnormalities. Congenital abnormalities, such as ventricular septal defect, sacral agenesis and hypoplastic left colon occur more frequently.

54 A = False   **B** = False   **C** = True   **D** = True   **E** = False

X-LINKED HYPOGAMMAGLOBULINAEMIA
These patients generally develop symptoms at around 4 months when the level of maternal IgG falls. Splenomegaly is not a feature but paucity of lymphoid tissue such as nodes and tonsils is. Pulmonary infection is common and requires aggressive management to prevent the development of bronchiectasis. Although pyogenic bacteria are the most common infecting organisms these patients may develop echovirus encephalitis. Management is with regular intravenous immunoglobulin infusions not bone marrow transplant.

55 A = False   **B** = True   **C** = True   **D** = True   **E** = False

Duchenne muscular dystrophy which is inherited as an X-linked recessive, may present with mental handicap although it more often presents with a delay in walking, a waddling gait, difficulty in climbing stairs and difficulty rising from the prone position (Gower sign). Creatinine kinase is grossly elevated from birth. Boys lose the ability to walk by the age of 12 and most die before the age of 20.

56 A = False   **B** = False   **C** = False   **D** = True   **E** = False

Juvenile chronic arthritis (JCA) is defined as chronic arthritis developing before 16 years and present for more than 3 months with the exclusion of other diseases. Only 20% have a systemic onset while 65% have a pauci-articular onset (involving less than five joints). Tests for rheumatoid factor are positive in a small minority, usually in girls who have juvenile rheumatoid disease but anti-nuclear antibody is often present in pauci-articular chronic juvenile arthritis and ANCA indicates a significant risk of chronic uveitis. The long-term prognosis for juvenile chronic arthritis is good with most children leading normal adult lives.

57 **A** = False   **B** = True   **C** = True   **D** = True   **E** = True

Cows' milk protein intolerance which may follow gastroenteritis usually presents with gastrointestinal symptoms such as diarrhoea and vomiting. Wheezing alone is a rare symptom. RAST to cow's milk or skin tests to cows' milk are often negative. A small intestinal biopsy may show partial villous atrophy which is less severe than that seen in coeliac disease.

58 **A** = True   **B** = False   **C** = True   **D** = True   **E** = False

Congenital hypothyroidism is most often due to thyroid dysgenesis but may occasionally be a transient phenomenon. Although detection by neonatal screening has greatly improved the prognosis, a small deficit in IQ is probably inevitable as a result of prenatal thyroxine deficiency.

59 **A** = True   **B** = True   **C** = False   **D** = False   **E** = False

Osteomyelitis most often involves the distal femur and the proximal tibia. The organism most often implicated is *Staphylococcus aureus* followed by *Haemophilus influenzae*. Radiological abnormalities do not appear until after the first week. Antibiotics should be given for 6 weeks.

60 **A** = False   **B** = False   **C** = True   **D** = False   **E** = False

Physiological jaundice is common and affects almost half of all newborn babies. Jaundice during the first 24 to 48 hours of life should be regarded as being due to haemolysis – usually ABO or rhesus incompatibility. Persistence of jaundice for 2 to 3 weeks may sometimes occur in normal babies, especially if breast-fed but underlying disorders should be considered. It is especially important in this situation to exclude conjugated hyperbilirubinamia. Pale stools suggest the presence of cholestasis.

TEST 2
Answers to Multiple-Choice Questions

1   **A** = False   **B** = True   **C** = True   **D** = True   **E** = True

The child development centre may be provided either in the hospital site or in the community. It provides both assessment and treatment for children with physical or mental disability, or for those with chronic illness. It should provide accommodation for the multidisciplinary team, including those from Education and Social Services, and the voluntary sector.

2   **A** = False   **B** = True   **C** = False   **D** = False   **E** = False

The philosophy of education for children with special educational needs has changed in recent years. Instead of different curricula for different children, the same curriculum (the National Curriculum) is provided for all children. However, it is recognised that different children require different methods, rates and levels of delivery according to their ability. Instead of placing children of different abilities in different classes (streaming), teachers are trained to teach mixed ability classes by 'differentiation' – to allow students in the same classroom to reach different achievement levels according to their individual ability. Teachers may do this by providing different resources to different children, by supporting individual children according to their needs, and by setting tasks so that the children may respond to them in different ways depending on their abilities. Children are no longer placed in schools depending on their diagnostic label (e.g. ESN(S) or ESN(M)), but according to their individual needs and the available resources of different schools. Children are integrated into normal schools whenever possible.

3   **A** = True   **B** = True   **C** = True   **D** = True   **E** = False

Day-care facilities may be provided by childminders, playgroups, day nurseries or family centres. Day nurseries are mostly run by social services departments, although they may also be run privately or by voluntary organisations. They are required to be registered and approved by the social services departments, and they should be staffed by qualified nursery nurses. Playgroups are for pre-school children, and they are run by trained playgroup leaders. They must be approved and registered with the local authority. Family centres are usually attended by both children and their parents, and they aim to improve the parenting skills of the parents and the confidence of the parents in managing their children.

4   **A** = False   **B** = False   **C** = False   **D** = True   **E** = True

The number of adoptions has been decreasing since the 1970s. Adoptions can be made usually through an authorised adoption agency, except when the prospective adopter is a relative. The minimum age of prospective adopters is

21. This is reduced to 18 if the adopters are the child's parent and step-parent. In considering applications for adoptions, adoption agencies must regard the welfare of the children as paramount. People who were adopted have a right of access to their original birth certificates after the age of 18 years.

5   **A** = True   **B** = True   **C** = False   **D** = False   **E** = False

Secondary prevention seeks to detect diseases at a presymptomatic stage so that their progress can be stopped and the harmful effects prevented. Galactosaemia can be detected by Guthrie's test neonatally, and congenital dislocation of the hips can be detected by neonatal examination. These are examples of secondary prevention. Immunisation against tetanus seeks to prevent the disease in the first place, and is an example of primary prevention. Enforcing the law on seat-belts for children is an example of prevention by health protection. In tertiary prevention, the aim is to minimise complications from established disease. Stabilising brittle diabetes is an example of tertiary prevention.

6   **A** = False   **B** = False   **C** = False   **D** = True   **E** = True

Regular routine physical examinations by the school doctors and examination of all students at entrance were practised in the past, with no evidence that they were effective. Selective but more detailed medical examination for those children who cause concern to parents or teachers is more effective. Examination should ideally be performed in a private room in the school. There should be a named nurse and doctor for every school, who are readily accessible to children and parents. There should also be a good working relationship between teachers and the school health team.

7   **A** = True   **B** = True   **C** = False   **D** = True   **E** = False

Measles, mumps, rubella, diphtheria, whooping cough and tetanus, which the child can be protected against by immunisation, are notifiable. Other notifiable bacterial infections include meningococcal disease, food poisoning, and ophthalmia neonatorum. Tuberculosis is also notifiable.

8   **A** = True   **B** = True   **C** = False   **D** = True   **E** = True

Measles typically presents with a maculopapular rash which initially appears behind the ears and on the face, and spreads to the rest of the body. Koplik's spots characteristically appear shortly before the onset of the rash. Children may also have coryzal symptoms, dry cough and conjunctivitis. Complications include secondary chest infection, acute encephalitis and subacute sclerosing panencephalitis (SSPE). SSPE may occur many years after the initial infection.

9   **A** = True   **B** = False   **C** = True   **D** = True   **E** = True

Type B is the most invasive type of *Haemophilus influenzae*, and is encapsulated. It may cause chest infection, otitis media, epiglottitis and meningitis in children. It is the main cause of epiglottitis. *Haemophilus* meningitis has a high rate of neurological sequelae, including sensori-neural deafness and subdural collection. *Staphylococcus*, *Pseudomonas* and *Haemophilus influenzae* are the three most common pathogens in cystic fibrosis.

10 **A** = True   **B** = False   **C** = True   **D** = True   **E** = False

Toddler diarrhoea occurs in children between 1 and 3 years of age. The symptoms are passage of frequent loose stools with undigested particles without evidence of failure to thrive. Children who drink excessive amounts of fruit juices are more prone to develop it. No treatment is necessary. This is a totally benign condition, and the parents should be reassured.

11 **A** = False   **B** = False   **C** = True   **D** = True   **E** = False

There is currently no biochemical test which can diagnose growth retardation due to psychological deprivation, although increased growth when placed in a different environment strongly suggests the diagnosis. These children sometimes show a reduced growth hormone response to a stimulation test, which is reversible when they are moved to a better environment. The management of such children is often difficult, and much psychosocial support is required.

12 **A** = False   **B** = True   **C** = True   **D** = False   **E** = True

An average 18-month old child can go upstairs two feet per step with hand held, but cannot kick a ball until 2 years of age. He or she can build a tower of three cubes. He or she can wave bye-bye and show anxiety of strangers at 1 year of age.

13 **A** = False   **B** = False   **C** = False   **D** = False   **E** = False

Visual acuity should be regularly tested after school entry, as myopia may develop after school entry. A newborn baby can usually fixate on a large object, but is not able to follow a large object horizontally 180° until about 4 months of age. At 3 years of age, it is more reliable to use a linear Snellen chart than single letters. This is due to 'crowding phenomenon', when single letters are seen more easily than a row of letters.

14 **A** = False   **B** = True   **C** = True   **D** = False   **E** = True

Clumsy children have problems of motor coordination usually without other developmental problems. The condition may affect up to 10% of all children. It should not include those with specific neurological conditions such as cerebellar ataxia or cerebral palsy. It affects both fine and gross motor skills. The aetiology is unclear. Children should be managed by a multidisciplinary team consisting of a paediatrician, educational psychologist, occupational therapist and physio-therapist.

15 **A** = False   **B** = True   **C** = True   **D** = False   **E** = False

In general, a child with a history of accidental poisoning within the previous 4 hours should have vomiting induced with ipecacuanha. However, if the substance ingested is volatile (e.g. petrol), there is a danger of inhalation causing pneumonitis. Also, if a corrosive substance has been ingested, induced vomiting may damage the oesophagus. In these cases, ipecacuanha should not be given. Aspirin and tricyclic antidepressants delay gastric emptying, and ipecacuanha can be given even if more than 4 hours have elapsed.

16 A = True   **B** = False   **C** = False   **D** = True   **E** = True

Meningitis is more difficult to diagnose in infants than in older children. The symptoms are usually non-specific and include irritability, refusal to feed, vomiting, lethargy and crying when handled. The signs are also non-specific and include a bulging fontanelle, irritability, and looking unwell. Convulsions may occur. Projectile vomiting is a sign of pyloric stenosis.

17 A = True   **B** = True   **C** = True   **D** = True   **E** = True

The majority of girls with Turner's syndrome have XO karyotype. In the neonatal period, they may have oedema of the hands and feet. In childhood, they characteristically have short stature, short webbed neck, low hairline, widely spaced nipples and wide carrying angles at the elbow (cubitus valgus). In addition, they may have pigmented naevi, and short fourth metacarpals. They may have coarctation of the aorta, and more than 30% have underlying renal abnormalities such as horseshoe kidneys. They may have hypertension resulting either from coarctation of the aorta or renal abnormalities. They usually have primary amenorrhoea (except mosaic Turner's XX/XO, when they may have periods for a few cycles), and are therefore infertile. The average IQ is about 90–95, and most of them have normal intellectual development.

18 A = True   **B** = True   **C** = True   **D** = False   **E** = True

Babies who are large for their gestational age are defined as babies heavier than the 90th centile for gestational age. They may be constitutionally large babies, or they may be infants of diabetic mothers or have other disorders such as Sotos syndrome (cerebral gigantism) or Beckwith's syndrome. They are more likely to suffer birth trauma and birth asphyxia due to their size. Infants of diabetic mothers may have other problems including hypoglycaemia, idiopathic respiratory distress syndrome, jaundice and polycythaemia.

19 A = False   **B** = False   **C** = True   **D** = False   **E** = False

Ophthalmia neonatorum (conjunctivitis within the first 28 days) is caused by *Chlamydia*, *Staphylococcus*, *Gonococcus*, herpes simplex virus, and other organisms. As some of the infections can be extremely serious, swabs must be taken for microbiological examination before treatment is started. Although the symptoms caused by *Chlamydia* can be mild, it can cause corneal scarring, and prompt treatment with both topical tetracycline and systemic erythromycin is required. *Gonococcus* is usually acquired during vaginal delivery, and usually presents in the first few days after birth, with copious discharge and conjunctival and lid oedema. Penetration of the cornea can occur causing blindness. Hence, both topical and systemic penicillin treatment must be started promptly.

20 **A** = True   **B** = True   **C** = False   **D** = False   **E** = False

There is a slight risk of a neurological reaction from pertussis immunisation, but the benefits outweigh the risks. Definite contraindications to pertussis immunisation include definite reaction to a previous dose, definite convulsion within 72 hours of immunisation, or progressive neurological disease. Hence, tuberous sclerosis is a contraindication. Prematurity and cystic fibrosis are not contraindications to immunisation. As pertussis vaccine is a killed vaccine, infants who are immunocompromised or taking steroids may receive pertussis vaccination.

21 **A** = True   **B** = False   **C** = False   **D** = True   **E** = False

An average infant has full head control at 20 weeks. A 6-month old infant can grasp an object with the palm, but will not have an index approach until 9 months. He or she cannot stand holding on to furniture or play 'pat-a-cake' until 12 months of age.

22 **A** = True   **B** = True   **C** = False   **D** = False   **E** = True

Cows' milk protein intolerance usually develops in the first 6 months, and affects mainly bottle-fed babies. However, breast-fed babies are not totally immune, as cows' milk protein may be secreted in the mother's milk if her diet contains cows' milk. An increased IgE level, high eosinophil count, or positive RAST tests to cows' milk may be present in some cases. As the condition improves with a cows' milk free diet, and is self-limiting, jejunal biopsy is only required in those who fail to respond to an exclusion diet. Dieticians should always be involved in supervising the diet.

23 **A** = True   **B** = False   **C** = True   **D** = True   **E** = True

Hirschsprung's disease is divided into the long-segment or the short-segment type depending on the length of aganglionic segment. The 'short-segment' type affects the rectum and sigmoid colon only, while the 'long-segment' type affects the bowel above the sigmoid colon. The 'long-segment' type presents in the first few days of life with failure to pass meconium, abdominal distension, and vomiting; and may present with life-threatening enterocolitis. The 'short-segment' type may present later with chronic constipation. A definitive diagnosis can be obtained by rectal biopsy.

24 **A** = False   **B** = False   **C** = False   **D** = True   **E** = False

More than 10% of children in United Kingdom have asthma to some extent. Both the severity and prevalence of asthma have increased over the last 20 years. The reasons for this are not entirely clear. The mortality rate for asthma has not declined in the last 10 years. More children are admitted to hospital than before. However, this may be due to increased awareness amongst parents and clinicians rather than a true increase in the prevalence. Although bronchiolitis in infancy is more common in winter, asthma is less troublesome in winter than in other parts of the year. Nocturnal cough is a common symptom of asthma in children.

25 A = False **B** = True **C** = False **D** = True **E** = True

Beclomethasone can be given via an inhaler, but nebulised beclomethasone is not available. Budesonide may be given via a nebuliser. The slight risk of oral candidiasis may be minimised by using a spacer device and by washing out the mouth afterwards. If steroids need to be given systemically, alternate day oral steroids are preferable to daily oral steroids, and less growth suppressing. As steroids affect glucose tolerance, urine should be regularly checked for glucose to detect glycosuria.

26 A = True **B** = True **C** = True **D** = True **E** = False

Ninety-five per cent of children with cystic fibrosis have pancreatic insufficiency resulting in steatorrhoea. They are more prone to chest infections, especially by *Staphylococcus*, *Haemophilus influenzae* and *Pseudomonas*. They typically develop bronchiectasis, and have clubbing of the fingers. While 8% of children develop diabetes mellitus later in life, it is not a characteristic feature of the disease.

27 A = True **B** = False **C** = True **D** = False **E** = False

Viral croup is most often caused by parainfluenza virus, followed by respiratory syncytial virus and rhinovirus. Viral croup affects mainly children aged 3 or under. Coryzal symptoms are followed by a dry harsh barking cough. Inspiratory stridor develops, which is worse at night and on exertion. Most cases are self-limiting; a minority progress to severe airway obstruction. Signs of severe airway obstruction include irritability, tachycardia, tachypnoea, cyanosis, and intercostal or subcostal recession.

28 A = False **B** = False **C** = True **D** = True **E** = False

In patent ductus arteriosus, there is a left to right shunt from the aorta to the pulmonary artery. The pulse is prominent or collapsing, with a wide pulse pressure. Patients with aortic incompetence (regurgitation) have a widened pulse pressure, left ventricular apical impulse, and a blowing high-pitched early diastolic murmur. Aortic stenosis causes a narrow pulse pressure. In coarctation of the aorta, the femoral pulses are absent or in older children weak with radio-femoral delay. The pulses in the upper limbs are usually normal. In congestive heart failure, the pulse is weak.

29 A = False **B** = True **C** = False **D** = True **E** = True

The incidence of congenital heart disease is about 8 per 1000 live births. The incidence of acyanotic heart disease is at least three times that of cyanotic heart disease. Ventricular septal defect is the most common acyanotic heart lesion, followed by patent ductus arteriosus and pulmonary stenosis. Fallot's tetralogy and transposition of the great arteries are the most common cyanotic heart lesions. Most cyanotic lesions require surgical intervention, and acyanotic lesions generally have a better prognosis than cyanotic lesions.

30 A = True   **B** = True   **C** = True   **D** = False   **E** = False

There are two main types of coarctation of the aorta, depending on the position of the constriction in relation to the ductus. The preductal type usually presents in the neonatal period with acute onset of shock when the ductus closes. Those with less obstruction may be asymptomatic in childhood, and a murmur or hypertension may be detected in adulthood. Characteristically, the femoral pulses are weak, and there is significant radio-femoral delay in later childhood. There is often an ejection systolic murmur at the left sternal edge radiating to the back between the scapulae. Coarctation should be corrected surgically to prevent the risks of hypertension and infective endocarditis.

31 A = True   **B** = True   **C** = True   **D** = False   **E** = False

Hydrocephalus may be due to increased production of cerebrospinal fluid (CSF), obstruction to the CSF flow, or decreased absorption from the arachnoid villi. Increased production may rarely be due to a choroid plexus tumour. Obstruction to the CSF flow may occur at the outlet of the fourth ventricle, in which case non-communicating hydrocephalus results. Examples are cerebellar tumours or tumours near to the ventricular systems, or stenosis of the aqueduct of Sylvius. Alternatively, obstruction may occur at the subarachnoid spaces, in which case communicating hydrocephalus results. Meningitis especially in the neonatal period may cause increased fibrin deposition which blocks the arachnoid granulations causing communicating hydrocephalus. While cerebral palsy may be associated with hydrocephalus, it is not the direct cause.

32 A = True   **B** = True   **C** = False   **D** = True   **E** = True

The first step in the management of status epilepticus is to check the airway, breathing and circulation, and to administer oxygen. Blood glucose should be checked to detect hypoglycaemia. Rectal or intravenous diazepam is the usual first-line treatment. Intramuscular paraldehyde may be given if diazepam is ineffective. The next line of treatment is intravenous phenytoin which must be given slowly under ECG control. If this is ineffective, mannitol infusion to reduce cerebral oedema, intravenous chlormethiazole, or general anaesthesia should be considered.

33 A = True   **B** = False   **C** = True   **D** = True   **E** = False

The first-line drug treatment is early analgesia (e.g. paracetamol). Aspirin is avoided in children under the age of 12 because of an association with Reye's syndrome. If attacks become frequent and severe, prophylactic treatment with propranolol or pizotifen can be tried. Avoidance of triggering factors (e.g. foods) is sometimes helpful.

34 A = True   **B** = True   **C** = True   **D** = False   **E** = True

Congenital abnormalities involving the posterior fossa such as the Dandy–Walker syndrome result in ataxia. Posterior fossa tumours such as medulloblastoma should always be excluded in the recent onset of ataxia. Acute cerebellar ataxia which occurs usually in pre-school children may follow viral infections such as chickenpox or echovirus. Anticonvulsants particularly phenytoin can cause ataxia. The Guillian–Barré syndrome causes symmetrical weakness and not ataxia.

35 **A** = True **B** = False **C** = True **D** = False **E** = True

Glandular fever, or infectious mononucleosis, is caused by Epstein–Barr virus. It is usually transmitted by direct contact, although it can be transmitted by droplets. It affects children and young adults. Patients have pyrexia, sore throat, marked enlargement of cervical lymph nodes, and general malaise. They may have associated mild splenomegaly. Haematological features include lymphocytosis and atypical lymphocytes. The Paul–Bunnell test may be negative in glandular fever in the early stages of the disease.

36 **A** = False **B** = True **C** = True **D** = False **E** = True

Accidents and congenital abnormalities are the most common causes of death in children. Leukaemia constitutes about one-third of all malignancies, and is the most common form of childhood cancer followed by brain tumour which is the most common solid tumour in childhood. While environmental factors such as radiation have been shown to be important in some specific cases, they are not a major cause of leukaemia. Viruses such as Epstein–Barr or HTLV viruses are recognised causes of childhood cancers.

37 **A** = False **B** = True **C** = True **D** = True **E** = True

Nephrotic syndrome is due to minimal change glomerulonephritis in the majority of the cases. These children have the best prognosis, and usually respond well to prednisolone therapy. Characteristic features of nephrotic syndrome include oedema, proteinuria, hypoalbuminaemia, and hyperlipidaemia. It is about twice as common in boys as in girls.

38 **A** = True **B** = True **C** = True **D** = True **E** = False

Tall stature may be constitutional, with the height similar to the mid-parental height centiles; hormonal (due to early puberty, hyperthyroidism or excessive growth hormone production); or caused by syndromes (such as Marfan's syndrome and Klinefelter's syndrome). Turner's syndrome presents with short stature.

39 **A** = True **B** = True **C** = False **D** = False **E** = False

Insulin is usually given twice daily before meals in the morning and evening, although a once daily regime may be sufficient in the 'honeymoon period'. Usually, two-thirds of the total insulin are given in the morning, and one-third in the evening. About one-third of the insulin should be short-acting. Absorption is faster if given subcutaneously in the abdomen rather than in the thigh, and in the thigh rather than in the arm. In an alternative regime, a long-acting insulin is given once daily and a pen injector which delivers short-acting insulin is given before meals.

40 A = False   **B** = False   **C** = True   **D** = True   **E** = True

Pertussis affects children of all age groups including neonates, as there is little passive protection from maternal antibodies. Infants are more severely affected, sometimes with apnoea attacks. It affects girls more than boys. The incubation period is about 7 to 14 days. The disease usually begins with the catarrhal phase with pyrexia, rhinorrhea and dry cough and then enters the paroxysmal phase with bouts of coughing ending with a whoop on inspiration, or with vomiting. Paroxysmal cough may lead to venous congestion and subconjunctival haemorrhages. The convalescent phase may take many months.

41 A = True   **B** = False   **C** = False   **D** = True   **E** = True

Congenital dislocation of the hips is more common in those with a positive family history, girls, white people, and those born by breech delivery. The condition can be diagnosed clinically by the Ortolani's or Barlow's test. Ultrasound examination has proved effective in diagnosing the condition without risk of radiation.

42 A = False   **B** = True   **C** = True   **D** = True   **E** = False

Sickle-cell anaemia results from substitution of one amino acid (valine for glutamine in position 6) of the globin chain of haemoglobin. This predisposes to aggregation in the deoxygenated state with distortion of the red cell envelope causing sickling. It seldom presents before the age of 6 months, because of the presence of foetal haemoglobin. Patients may present with painful crises, with pain and swelling of the small bones ('the hand–foot syndrome') triggered by infection or dehydration. Patients may also present with aplastic crises, or with *Pneumococcus* or *Salmonella* infection. Polyuria may occur in later childhood because of renal tubular damage. Mild to moderate splenomegaly is common in early childhood, but rare thereafter because splenic infarcts cause autosplenectomy.

43 A = True   **B** = True   **C** = False   **D** = True   **E** = False

Features of rickets in infancy include a large anterior fontanelle whose closure is often delayed, craniotabes, enlargement of costochondral junctions (rachitic rosary), and swelling of the wrists and ankles. Toddlers may have genu varum and older children genu valgum. Bleeding gums is a feature of scurvy rather than rickets.

44 A = False   **B** = True   **C** = False   **D** = True   **E** = True

The Moro reflex, one of the primitive reflexes, usually disappears at 3 to 4 months of age. Its persistence at 7 months would suggest a serious neurodevelopmental problem. The normal 6-month old can transfer objects from hand to hand and can roll over but crawling forwards is not achieved until 9 months. Some normal babies progress by shuffling and do not crawl until well into the second year. Most babies start to laugh at about 4 months.

45 A = True   **B** = True   **C** = True   **D** = False   **E** = True

The possibility of hypothyroidism should be borne in mind in a young child with Down's syndrome who seems very developmentally delayed or in the older child whose growth is falling off. Duodenal atresia is the most common gastro-intestinal malformation. Sensori-neural deafness and secretory otitis media are common in children with trisomy 21. The incidence of leukaemia in childhood is increased. Also, neonates with trisomy 21 sometimes have a leukaemoid reaction in the blood which may spontaneously regress.

46 A = False   **B** = True   **C** = False   **D** = False   **E** = False

Hereditary spherocytosis, which has an autosomal dominant inheritance, is more common in people of Northern European descent. Severe neonatal jaundice may occur with its onset in the first 24 hours of life. Laboratory features include anaemia, the prevalence of spherocytes on blood film and increased osmotic fragility. A splenectomy should be postponed until later childhood or adolescence because of the risk of infection although it is occasionally required earlier in severely affected children.

47 A = True   **B** = False   **C** = True   **D** = False   **E** = True

Growth hormone deficiency may present with hypoglycaemia and small external genitalia in male infants who are usually of normal birth weight. As well as being small, affected children are often overweight and appear young for their age (cherubic appearance). Before puberty, body proportions are normal.

48 A = True   **B** = True   **C** = True   **D** = False   **E** = True

Incomplete bladder emptying and constipation encourage urine stasis, which predisposes to infection. Bubble bath may facilitate the entry of bacteria into the urethra. Myelomeningocoele is often associated with a neuropathic bladder.

49 A = False   **B** = True   **C** = False   **D** = False   **E** = True

Slipped upper femoral epiphysis, which may be bilateral in about one-third of cases, is more common in boys. The condition usually occurs in later childhood or adolescence and presents with pain and difficulty walking. Premature degen-erative arthritis may occur in adult life.

50 A = False   **B** = False   **C** = True   **D** = True   **E** = False

Breast development without other signs of puberty occurs in girls before the age of 3 years and is a benign condition, usually regressing within 2 years. There is often isolated ovarian cyst development. Growth velocity and bone age are normal. Observation alone is required to ensure that other signs of precocious puberty do not develop.

51 A = False   **B** = True   **C** = True   **D** = False   **E** = True

A fractured clavicle in a 2-week old baby is likely to have occurred at birth.

Metaphyseal and epiphyseal fractures are typical of non-accidental injury and are due to twisting and pulling injuries. Rib fractures in the absence of major trauma (e.g. a road traffic accident) and bone disease are pathognomonic for abuse in young children. Single linear parietal fractures have a low specificity whereas bilateral skull fractures and depressed skull fractures especially of the occiput have a high specificity for abuse.

52 **A** = False   **B** = True   **C** = True   **D** = True   **E** = False

In addition to heavy proteinuria, about 25% of patients have transient microscopic haematuria. Gross haematuria raises the possibility of pathology other than minimal change glomerulonephritis and indicates the need for a renal biopsy. Children with the nephrotic syndrome are vulnerable to infection. *Streptococcus pneumoniae* can cause peritonitis and septicaemia and oedematous children with ascites should receive penicillin. Abdominal pain is not uncommon in the nephrotic child but may indicate peritonitis or hypovolaemia. In the latter, there is evidence of peripheral circulatory failure and treatment with plasma or albumin is required. Over 75% of patients will subsequently relapse and up to 50% will relapse frequently.

53 **A** = False   **B** = False   **C** = True   **D** = False   **E** = True

Systemic steroids are ineffective in bronchiolitis and antibiotics should not be given. Respiratory syncytial virus (RSV) infection may present with apnoeic episodes in ex-preterm babies. Droplet spread is common and measures should be taken to protect other infants. As many as 75% of children have further episodes of wheeze in the following 2 years.

54 **A** = True   **B** = False   **C** = True   **D** = True   **E** = False

Types I and IV osteogenesis imperfecta are inherited as autosomal dominant while the more severe Type III in which features are often present at birth is inherited as autosomal recessive. Osteogenesis imperfecta is due to abnormal collagen synthesis. Short stature is common, but hearing impairment occurs in adults with the condition.

55 **A** = True   **B** = False   **C** = True   **D** = True   **E** = False

Giardiasis varies from being asymptomatic to producing severe diarrhoea and malabsorption. Blood and mucous are absent from the stools. One should consider the possibility of immunodeficiency in patients with giardiasis. Cysts may be difficult to find in the stools. Examination of duodenal juice or small intestinal mucosa for trophozoites is more reliable.

56 **A** = False   **B** = True   **C** = False   **D** = True   **E** = True

The presence of splenomegaly in children with thrombocytopenia would suggest diagnoses other than idiopathic thrombocytopenic purpura. The initial presentation of symptomatic HIV positive children often includes lymphadenopathy, splenomegaly, fever and failure to thrive. In addition to hepatomegaly and conjugated hyperbilirubinaemia, patients with neonatal hepatitis frequently have splenomegaly. A number of storage diseases (e.g. Gaucher's disease, Niemann–Pick disease and mucopolysaccharidosis) also cause splenomegaly.

57 A = True   **B** = True   **C** = False   **D** = False   **E** = True

Acute idiopathic thrombocytopenic purpura (ITP) is essentially a benign condition with a low risk of serious bleeding such as intracranial haemorrhage. Thus, no treatment is a therapeutic option. Corticosteroids cause a faster recovery of platelet count but bone marrow examination is essential before administration to exclude leukaemia. Failure to do so may delay diagnosis of leukaemia and jeopardise survival. Intravenous immunoglobulin may be effective but has potential side-effects. Platelet infusion is only given if life threatening haemorrhage occurs. This is a rare event.

58 A = False   **B** = True   **C** = True   **D** = False   **E** = True

The floppy infant syndrome may be caused by disorders of the CNS (e.g. perinatal hypoxia), connective tissue disorders, metabolic disorders, the Prader–Willi syndrome (hypotonia, hypogonadism and obesity), spinal cord disorders (e.g. spinal cord injury), Werdnig–Hoffmann disease, hereditary neuropathies and hereditary myopathies.

59 A = False   **B** = True   **C** = True   **D** = True   **E** = False

In vitamin D deficiency, serum calcium concentrations are normal or low, phosphate levels are low and alkaline phosphatase activity is elevated. Clinical features include metaphyseal flaring, prominence of costochondrial junctions, frontal bossing, genu valgum, bowing of the tibia and bone pain in older children. X-rays reveal widened frayed metaphyses and generalised bone demineralisation.

60 A = True   **B** = False   **C** = False   **D** = False   **E** = True

In the United Kingdom, the majority of cases are caused by Group B meningococci to which an effective vaccine is not available, although the proportion of cases due to Group C has increased since 1995. Vaccines against Groups A and C are available, and may be given to travellers to regions where these strains are prevalent. Rifampicin is the antibiotic of choice for eradication of meningococci in household contacts, and for those who have had mouth-to-mouth contact. Benzylpenicillin should be given immediately by the first doctor to suspect meningococcal disease.

TEST 3
Answers to Multiple-Choice Questions

1 **A** = True   **B** = True   **C** = True   **D** = True   **E** = True

The planning of child health services requires the collection and analysis of information concerning the population needs for child health services, so that appropriate care may be commissioned by the purchasers. There should be collaboration between purchasers and providers to negotiate the appropriate contracts according to the assessed needs, and there should be collaboration among both professionals in the health service and professionals inside and outside the health service. Involvement of health services staff and managers is important.

2 **A** = False   **B** = False   **C** = True   **D** = True   **E** = True

In recent years, changes in the health services are mirrored in the educational sector. Just as general practitioners are encouraged to become fundholders, schools are encouraged to opt out of local authorities' control to become grant maintained, and take a more active part in the management of the school. Just as the views of patients are increasingly considered, parents are more involved in their children's education. Just as the cost effectiveness and performance of health services are increasingly monitored, the effectiveness of teaching in schools is also increasingly monitored. League tables according to examination results are published, and schools which consistently perform badly are threatened with closure.

3 **A** = False   **B** = False   **C** = False   **D** = False   **E** = True

Long-term fostering is used less frequently than previously, as adoption is thought to be a better alternative for long-term placement. Short-term fostering is seldom for more than 6 months. If more than 6 months' placement is required, adoption should be considered. Prospective foster carers may foster a maximum of three children, unless the children are siblings of a large family. Foster arrangements may be made by voluntary agencies, although local authorities must be satisfied that the arrangements are satisfactory. Foster parents are given detailed information about the child's health and development.

4 **A** = True   **B** = True   **C** = True   **D** = False   **E** = False

The composition and functions of the adoption panels are defined in the Adoption Agencies Regulations 1983. They consist of between 7 and 10 members, including two social workers employed by the Agency, a medical adviser, a management representative and two independent persons. A legal adviser is not a statutory requirement, although the panel would usually require legal advice. There must be at least one man and one woman.

5　**A** = False　**B** = True　**C** = True　**D** = False　**E** = True

The characteristic features of attention deficit disorder are early onset (usually below the age of 5), overactivity, inattention and inability to persist with a task. These features usually occur in different situations and over a period of time. Impaired attention and overactivity are necessary for the diagnosis to be made. Other features include recklessness, being prone to accidents, lack of social inhibition, cognitive impairment and sometimes specific motor or language disorders. The disorder tends to persist throughout the school years and sometimes into adulthood, although frequently, there is improvement in activity and attention.

6　**A** = False　**B** = False　**C** = True　**D** = True　**E** = False

Conduct disorders are characterised by antisocial or aggressive behaviour amounting to a major violation of age-appropriate social expectations. The behaviour must be repetitive and persistent (ICD 10 definition). Hence, they cannot be diagnosed from a single violent episode. Conduct disorders are the most common psychiatric disorders, especially in older children and adolescents. All studies show that they are more common in boys than girls. They are commonly associated with adverse psychological environments such as unsatisfactory family relationships at home. While persistent truancy and running away from home may constitute conduct disorders, persistent school refusal is usually an emotional disorder.

7　**A** = True　**B** = False　**C** = False　**D** = True　**E** = False

There are broadly three types of vaccines. Live vaccines include vaccines against mumps, rubella, measles and oral polio. Killed (inactivated) vaccines include vaccines against pertussis and *Haemophilus influenzae* Type B. Toxoids include vaccines against diphtheria and tetanus.

8　**A** = True　**B** = False　**C** = True　**D** = True　**E** = False

The MMR vaccine is a live vaccine which is given between the ages of 1 year to 18 months. A booster dose is also given at school entry. It should not be given before the age of 1 year, as the presence of maternal antibodies may prevent the child developing immunity. It may cause mild pyrexia a few days after the immunisation. Self-limiting aseptic meningitis may occur due to the mumps component. It is especially important to immunise children with cystic fibrosis, as they may develop secondary chest infection following measles.

9　**A** = False　**B** = False　**C** = True　**D** = True　**E** = True

Weaning is the change from a liquid diet of breast or bottle milk to feeding with a more varied diet. This change is a gradual process, and the exact time varies in different babies. Weaning usually occurs between the ages of 3 and 6 months. It should not be delayed as a milk diet alone does not contain sufficient nutrients for the infant to grow. The infant also requires iron from solids to replenish iron stored in the body.

10 **A** = False   **B** = True   **C** = False   **D** = True   **E** = True

Phenylketonurina is a metabolic problem due to deficiency of the enzyme phenylalanine hydroxylase which coverts phenylalanine to tyrosine. It is inherited as an autosomal recessive disorder. Neonatal screening uses the Guthrie or Scriver tests which detect increased blood phenylalanine level. It is important to detect the disease early, as brain damage occurs rapidly if children are not given a phenylalanine free diet. High phenylalanine levels during pregnancy may result in brain damage in the foetus.

11 **A** = False   **B** = True   **C** = True   **D** = True   **E** = True

Tall stature may be constitutional, caused by disease, or occur as part of a syndrome. Diseases causing tall stature include hypothalamic/pituitary disease or adrenal disease. Dysmorphic syndromes causing tall stature include Klinefelter syndrome, Marfan syndrome, and Sotos syndrome (cerebral gigantism). Russell–Silver syndrome is associated with short stature.

12 **A** = True   **B** = True   **C** = True   **D** = True   **E** = True

The average 3-year old can stand and walk on tip-toe, stand on one foot momentarily, and go upstairs one foot per step and downstairs two feet per step. He or she can copy a circle, but cannot copy a square until 4 years of age, and a triangle until 5 years of age.

13 **A** = False   **B** = True   **C** = True   **D** = False   **E** = False

Squints may be due to intraocular pathology such as retinoblastoma, and hence it is important to examine the fundus in any child presenting with a squint. However, most children do not have intraocular pathology, and squints are more often due to refractive errors (long- or short-sightedness, or astigmatism), or due to abnormal convergence to accommodation ratio. In an attempt to overcome double vision, children suppress vision in one eye, which may lead to amblyopia. In some types of squints, the child adopts an abnormal head posture to minimise the deviation of the affected eye. Alternating squints (when both eyes may be the 'seeing eye' at different times) are less likely to lead to amblyopia. Squints due to refractive errors and some types of squints due to abnormal convergence to accommodation ratio may be corrected by spectacles.

14 **A** = False   **B** = False   **C** = True   **D** = True   **E** = True

Most children with severe learning difficulties have a recognised cause. The most common cause is Down's syndrome, followed by neurological abnormalities and cerebral palsy. By contrast, most children with moderate learning difficulties have no recognised cause. Severe learning difficulties are more common in boys, partly due to the fragile X syndrome and sex-linked conditions. Children with severe learning difficulties may have intractable epilepsy and challenging behaviour, which make management difficult.

15 **A** = True   **B** = True   **C** = True   **D** = True   **E** = False

Tricyclic antidepressants may cause convulsions, loss of consciousness and agitation. Anticholinergic signs such as hot dry skin, dry mouth, dilated pupils, or tachycardia occur. Serious cardiac arrhythmias may be life-threatening. Children with a history of tricyclic antidepressants overdose should be admitted to hospital and observed closely including ECG monitoring for 48 hours.

16 **A** = True   **B** = False   **C** = False   **D** = True   **E** = True

Neisseria meningococcus is a Gram-negative diplococcus. *Meningococcus* usually causes septicaemia and/or meningitis in children. It can occasionally cause arthritis. In the United Kingdom, Group B is more common than either Group A and Group C. If a child has proven meningococcal disease, household and other close contacts in the 5 days prior to the onset of illness should be given prophylactic rifampicin. Vaccines are currently only available for Group A and Group C, but not for Group B. Adrenal haemorrhage may occur, which is rapidly fatal.

17 **A** = True   **B** = False   **C** = True   **D** = False   **E** = False

The fragile X syndrome is due to fragile sites on the X chromosomes, and is associated with moderate to severe mental retardation. The children characteristically have a long face, prominent jaw, large ears and large testes, but changes may be subtle or minimal. Their language and speech development are particularly affected. They have a higher incidence of associated autism. Some female heterozygotes show physical features. A minority have intellectual impairment.

18 **A** = False   **B** = True   **C** = True   **D** = True   **E** = True

Idiopathic respiratory distress syndrome, also known as hyaline membrane disease, is caused by surfactant deficiency, and affects mainly preterm babies. The deficiency of surfactant results in poor lung compliance, ventilation–perfusion mismatch, hypoxaemia and acidosis. Clinical features include cyanosis due to hypoxaemia, tachypnoea (more than about 55 per minute), sternal and intercostal recession. Chest X-ray in mild to moderate disease usually shows mottling with air bronchogram, but total 'white-out' in severe disease.

19 **A** = True   **B** = True   **C** = True   **D** = True   **E** = False

Rubella infection in the first trimester can cause the congenital rubella syndrome in the foetus with deafness, cataract, microophthalmia, microcephaly, congenital heart disease (patent ductus arteriosus or peripheral pulmonary stenosis), and hepatosplenomegaly. Human immunodeficiency virus can be transmitted to the foetus, with intrauterine growth retardation, hepatosplenomegaly, and microcephaly. Chickenpox acquired in the first trimester may cause abortion, or limb/cerebral abnormalities in the baby. If the mother is infected with chickenpox a few days before delivery, the baby can be severely affected with vesicles and pneumonitis. Cytomegalovirus can be transmitted to the baby causing microcephaly and retinopathy. Although *Toxoplasma* can be transmitted vertically, it is a protozoa and not a virus.

20 A = False **B** = False **C** = False **D** = True **E** = True

Definite contraindications to measles immunisation include immunodeficiency or immunosuppressive treatment, having received a live vaccine in the last 3 weeks, or untreated tuberculosis. Cerebral palsy is a non-progressive neurological disorder, and is not *per se* a contraindication. The clinical features of each child should be considered individually.

21 A = True **B** = False **C** = True **D** = True **E** = True

An average 3-year old child can go up stairs one foot per step and down stairs two feet per steps. He or she can momentarily stand on one foot. The child can copy a circle, but will not be able to copy a square until about 4 years of age, and a triangle until about the age of 5, and can give his or her full name and sex. He or she is usually dry by day and night before the age of 3, although 10% of children have nocturnal enuresis at 5 years of age.

22 A = True **B** = True **C** = False **D** = True **E** = True

Cystic fibrosis is the most common autosomal recessive disorder in the United Kingdom, and affects about 1 in every 2000 live births. It is less common in black Africans, and is very rare in the Chinese. The gene has been located to the long arm of chromosome 7. Pancreatic insufficiency may cause fat malabsorption and deficiencies of fat-soluble vitamins (i.e. vitamins A, D, E and K).

23 A = False **B** = True **C** = True **D** = False **E** = True

Children with toddler diarrhoea have loose stools of variable frequency and consistency often containing undigested food. These children are usually aged between 1 and 5 years, and are otherwise well and thrive normally. The mechanisms are poorly understood and the condition resolves spontaneously.

24 A = True **B** = True **C** = True **D** = False **E** = True

The most common trigger for reversible airway disease in infants is virus infection, often respiratory syncytial virus. In young children, viral infections often induce recurrent wheezy episodes, often labelled as wheezy bronchitis. Affected older children often, though not necessarily, have an atopic tendency, and a raised IgE level. Most affected children who develop asthma present before they are 5 years of age. In many children, asthma resolves spontaneously in adulthood and those who continue to have asthma as adults often have less severe symptoms.

25 A = False **B** = True **C** = False **D** = False **E** = False

The MMR vaccine contains live attenuated organisms. Tetanus and diphtheria immunisation contain inactivated toxins of tetanus and diphtheria toxoid. Pertussis vaccine contains killed *Bordetella pertussis* organisms. Pneumococcal vaccine contains a capsular polysaccharide extract of 23 subtypes of *Streptococcus pneumoniae*.

26 **A** = False   **B** = True   **C** = False   **D** = True   **E** = True

Children with cystic fibrosis have pancreatic insufficiency, resulting in malabsorption, especially of fat. A high calorie diet with a normal protein, carbohydrate and fat content should be given. Pancreatic enzyme supplements are taken prior to meals and snacks. There is a deficiency of fat-soluble vitamins (vitamin C is a water-soluble vitamin). Chest physiotherapy and postural drainage are important in the prevention and treatment of chest infection, and prophylactic flucloxacillin is useful in preventing staphylococcal chest infection.

27 **A** = True   **B** = False   **C** = True   **D** = True   **E** = False

Although respiratory syncytial virus is responsible for the majority of cases of bronchiolitis, other viruses such as rhinovirus can be responsible. Bronchiolitis usually presents before 9 months of age, and has a peak incidence at about 3 months. The severity of the illness is increased by cigarette smoke in the household. Infants may present with poor feeding due to dyspnoea. There is no restriction on ambient oxygen concentration.

28 **A** = False   **B** = False   **C** = True   **D** = True   **E** = True

A respiratory rate of 45 breaths per minute and pulse rate of 130 per minute in a 1-month old infant are within normal limits. Heart failure at this age often presents with poor feeding. Enlarged liver and gallop rhythm are physical signs of heart failure.

29 **A** = False   **B** = True   **C** = True   **D** = True   **E** = False

Ventricular septal defect is the most common congenital heart defect. The time of presentation depends on the size of the defect. Small defects are often asymptomatic and are detected on routine examination. Large defects may present in the first three months of life with failure to thrive and heart failure. Ventricular septal defect does not present at birth because the pulmonary vascular resistance prevents left to right shunting. Clinical examination may reveal an enlarged heart with thrusting apex due to left ventricular hypertrophy. There is characteristically a harsh pansystolic murmur loudest at the left lower sternal edge, often accompanied by a thrill. Most small defects close spontaneously, and do not require surgical treatment.

30 **A** = False   **B** = True   **C** = True   **D** = False   **E** = True

The four cardinal features of Fallot's tetralogy are ventricular septal defect, pulmonary stenosis, overriding of the aorta over the ventricular septum and resulting right ventricular hypertrophy. The degree of cyanosis depends on the severity of the pulmonary stenosis. Severe pulmonary stenosis causes severe obstruction to the right ventricular outflow tract which causes significant right to left shunt across the ventricular septum, resulting in cyanosis.

31 **A** = False   **B** = True   **C** = False   **D** = False   **E** = True

Febrile convulsions are the most common form of seizures in children, and occur in up to 5% of children. They affect children between 6 months and 5 years of age with a peak incidence during the first half of the second year, and are slightly more common in boys. There is often a positive family history. Convulsions are thought to be associated with a rapid increase in temperature, and commonly occur in the first 24 hours of a febrile illness.

32 A = True   **B** = False   **C** = True   **D** = True   **E** = True

Complex partial seizures account for about 20–30% of childhood seizures. They are sometimes associated with brain lesions such as previous ischaemic damage, infection, trauma or tumour and present with both motor and affective features. There may be an aura with altered sensation, *déjà vu* or hallucinations in any modalities (e.g. auditory, visual or olfactory). The features include impairment of consciousness, automatism such as lip smacking, chewing, pulling at clothing and sometimes a tonic-clonic seizure. Learning disorders and behavioural problems may be associated. Carbamazepine is the initial drug of choice.

33 A = True   **B** = False   **C** = False   **D** = True   **E** = False

Duchenne muscular dystrophy, the most common type of muscular dystrophy, is sex-linked recessive in inheritance. The gene responsible for the disease produces a protein called dystrophin, and children with Duchenne muscular dystrophy have low levels. It usually presents before the age of 5 years with frequent falls and difficulty in climbing stairs. Boys with Duchenne muscular dystrophy have a very high creatinine phosphokinase level which can be used as a screening test. It may be associated with cardiomyopathy and mental retardation.

34 A = False   **B** = True   **C** = True   **D** = False   **E** = True

Sensori-neural deafness in children may be congenital or acquired. Congenital causes include single gene inherited disorders (which may be autosomal dominant, autosomal recessive, or sex-linked recessive) as well as a number of syndromes. Prenatally acquired causes are usually due to maternal drugs or infection (e.g. rubella) in pregnancy. Other acquired causes include infections (e.g. *Haemophilus influenzae* infection, mumps), drugs (e.g. gentamicin), kernicterus, or rarely acoustic neuromas. Glue ear is a cause of conductive deafness. In elective mutism, the child refuses to speak, but hearing may be normal.

35 A = True   **B** = True   **C** = False   **D** = True   **E** = False

The aetiology of leukaemia is unknown in the majority of the cases. However, it is known that both genetic and environmental factors are important. Children with Down's syndrome have an increased risk of leukaemia. In the DNA repair deficiency syndromes such as Fanconi's anaemia and Bloom's syndrome, the risk of leukaemia is much increased. Radiation is known to increase the risk of leukaemia. Viruses such as Epstein–Barr virus are known to increase the risk of leukaemia. Leukaemia is more common in boys than in girls.

36 **A** = True   **B** = False   **C** = False   **D** = True   **E** = True

Urinary tract infections are more common in girls than in boys above the age of 1 year. In older children, urinary symptoms of dysuria and frequency are the most common presenting symptoms. In infancy, the presenting symptoms are usually non-specific with general malaise, pyrexia, and feeding problems. *E. coli* is responsible for about 90% of urinary tract infections. All children presenting with urinary tract infections for the first time should be investigated. Infants under the age of 1 year should have ultrasound, DMSA scan and micturating cystourethrogram; children between the ages of 1 and 5 should have ultrasound and DMSA scans, and those above the age of 5 years should have ultrasound performed.

37 **A** = True   **B** = True   **C** = True   **D** = True   **E** = True

Hypoalbuminaemia in the nephrotic syndrome may result in pleural effusion and ascites. Children with nephrotic syndrome are more likely to have infections, especially with *Pneumococcus* and Gram-negative bacteria. Hence, antibiotic prophylaxis with penicillin is recommended, and Pneumovax may be given in remission. The children are also more at risk of infective peritonitis both due to the ascites and to lowered resistance to infection. Nephrotic syndrome results in a low extracellular volume and a hypercoagulable state. Hence, they are at risk of both venous and arterial thrombosis, especially if they have hypovolaemia.

38 **A** = False   **B** = False   **C** = True   **D** = True   **E** = True

The most common cause of congenital hypothyroidism is thyroid dysgenesis. The thyroxine level is low, with a high TSH level due to lack of hypothalamic feedback inhibition. However, congenital hypothyroidism may rarely be due to pituitary deficiency resulting in low TSH as well as thyroxine levels. Screening tests for congenital hypothyroidism measure either thyroxine or TSH levels. In either case, the sensitivity is about 90%. Most cases of congenital hypothyroidism are detected by screening tests. Otherwise, children may present with poor feeding constipation, prolonged jaundice, or hypothermia. Significant developmental and intellectual deficits result if the treatment is delayed for more than a few weeks.

39 **A** = False   **B** = True   **C** = False   **D** = True   **E** = True

The diabetic child should be encouraged to take a diet containing low amounts of fat (to provide approximately 30% of the calorie requirement), adequate protein (about 15% of the calorie requirement) and carbohydrate (about 55% of the calorie requirement). Carbohydrate should be predominately derived from complex carbohydrates such as starch and highly refined sugars should be avoided. A high fibre content should be encouraged. Rotation of injection sites minimises the risk of lipoatrophy which can cause problems with control.

40 **A** = True   **B** = False   **C** = True   **D** = True   **E** = False

Measles is rare under 6 months of age since the infant has passive protection from maternal antibodies. It is highly infectious, and is mainly transmitted by droplets. The child usually has prodromal symptoms of coryza, conjunctivitis and a dry cough. Koplik's spots may be seen at this stage on the buccal mucosa. A maculo-papular rash then appears, initially behind the ears, and then spreads to the face and down the trunk. Post-infective neurological complications include post-infectious encephalomyelitis within 1 to 2 weeks after the infection. Subacute sclerosing panencephalitis, a rare complication, occurs many years later.

41   **A** = False   **B** = True   **C** = True   **D** = True   **E** = False

Strawberry naevi are capillary haemangiomas. They are not present at birth, but usually appear, in the first month or two of life, and then grow rapidly in infancy. They usually reach maximum size by about 1 year of age, and disappear spontaneously before 10 years of age. The majority involute before the child is 5 years old. Intradermal steroids or oral steroids may be tried if the haemangioma interferes with vital structures (e.g. an eyelid lesion interfering with vision). Laser therapy may also used. They may be complicated by ulceration or ulceration followed by infection. Bleeding occasionally occurs.

42   **A** = False   **B** = False   **C** = True   **D** = True   **E** = False

In beta thalassaemia major, there is impaired or absent production of beta globin chains. Affected children usually present in the first year of life with anaemia and failure to thrive. The blood picture shows a hypochromic microcytic anaemia, with a high reticulocyte count due to ineffective erythropoiesis. Children with beta thalassaemia major usually require regular blood transfusions. Some children with homozygous beta thalassaemia have thalassaemia intermedia and may not require transfusion. They must not be prescribed iron, as they are iron overloaded due to increased iron absorption and regular transfusions.

43   **A** = True   **B** = True   **C** = True   **D** = False   **E** = True

Henoch–Schönlein purpura is characterised by a purpuric rash affecting the legs, buttocks and extensor surfaces of the arms, gastro-intestinal symptoms (most commonly abdominal pain), arthritis and renal involvement. The latter usually consists of transient haematuria and proteinuria but chronic renal disease and nephrotic syndrome can occur. Gastrointestinal complications include haemorrhage, intussusception, obstruction and perforation. Angiooedema is common in younger children and may cause distressing scrotal oedema. Coronary artery aneurysms are a feature of Kawasaki syndrome.

44   **A** = False   **B** = True   **C** = False   **D** = True   **E** = True

Increased appetite is a common side-effect of sodium valproate but liver disease is rare and often very serious. Phenobarbitone, which is used less often nowadays, causes side-effects in about 25% of young children, particularly hyperactivity, irritability and drowsiness. Hirsutism occurs in some children taking phenytoin. Clonazepam may cause increased bronchial secretions which can be a problem especially in handicapped children.

45 **A** = False   **B** = False   **C** = False   **D** = False   **E** = True

Vomiting and allergic reactions are not contraindications to MMR immunisation, although it is prudent to immunise these children in a hospital setting. Boys with X-linked hypogammaglobulinaemia should not receive live vaccines although children with HIV infection may receive all routine immunisations except BCG and oral polio vaccines.

46 **A** = True   **B** = True   **C** = False   **D** = True   **E** = True

Children who drink excessive amount of orange squash may have diarrhoea as well as nutritional problems. Although most children with Hirschsprung's disease present in the neonatal period with delayed passage of meconium, abdominal distension and vomiting, later onset with overflow faecal soiling may occur. Children with severe combined immunodeficiency typically present with chronic diarrhoea, failure to thrive and respiratory infections.

47 **A** = False   **B** = False   **C** = True   **D** = True   **E** = True

Idiopathic respiratory distress syndrome (IRDS) is associated with decreased lung compliance. Pulmonary vasoconstriction contributes to right to left intra-pulmonary shunting and extrapulmonary (ductus arteriosus) shunting. IRDS is more common in infants of diabetic mothers, but heroin accelerates surfactant production in the foetus.

48 **A** = True   **B** = False   **C** = False   **D** = False   **E** = True

Breast milk jaundice is a common cause of prolonged unconjugated hyper-bilirubinaemia. Kernicterus does not occur and the condition is not an indication to stop breast feeding. It is important to exclude conjugated hyperbilirubinaemia in babies with prolonged jaundice as this may be due to neonatal hepatitis, cystic fibrosis or biliary atresia. Diagnosis of biliary atresia should be made before 6 weeks if surgical treatment is to be successful. Conjugated hyperbilirubinaemia does not cause kernicterus which is related to the level of free unconjugated bilirubin. In the Crigler–Najjar syndrome, persistently high unconjugated hyper-bilirubinaemia is due to deficiency of UDP-glucuronyl transferase.

49 **A** = False   **B** = True   **C** = True   **D** = True   **E** = True

IgA deficiency has an incidence of approximately 1 in 500 of the population and is often asymptomatic. Recurrent infection is more likely when associated with IgG_2 deficiency (the genes coding for IgG_2 and IgA are close together on chromosome 14). IgA deficiency is associated with an increased incidence of food allergy, atopy, coeliac disease and autoimmune disorders.

50 **A** = True   **B** = False   **C** = False   **D** = False   **E** = False

Splenomegaly is common in sickle-cell disease in the first few years of life, but becomes less common after 6 years of age as the spleen becomes pro-gressively fibrosed. Children with sickle-cell disease are very much at risk from infection and should be immunised against pneumococcus at 2 years of age (the vaccine is less effective before the age of 2 years) and receive long-term oral penicillin prophylaxis. The clinical course of the disease is better if HbF is high. Leg ulcers occur in adult sufferers of sickle-cell disease especially in the tropics.

51 A = True   B = False   C = True   D = False   E = True

Although many children with congenital cataract are otherwise healthy, there is a long list of potential causes including intrauterine infection, metabolic conditions (particularly galactosaemia), chromosome abnormalities and numerous syndromes. Subcapsular cataract may occur with prolonged use of steroids.

52 A = True   B = True   C = False   D = False   E = False

Human milk protein is approximately 60 to 70% whey and 30–40% casein. Human milk contains primarily saturated fat and less sodium and vitamin K than cows' milk.

53 A = False   B = True   C = True   D = True   E = True

Tension headache is the most common type of headache in children. Children with migraine often have a parent who is or has been similarly affected. Common triggers for migraine attacks include stress, fatigue, bright light, fasting and certain foods (e.g. cheese and chocolate). Transient ischaemic features such as hemiparesis, oculomotor paresis and sensory symptoms are uncommon but usually reversible.

54 A = False   B = True   C = True   D = False   E = False

The prognosis is worse for children aged less than 1 year or over 10 years. Among the prognostic factors indicating a worse prognosis are high white cell counts, low platelet counts, male sex and immunophenotype.

55 A = True   B = False   C = False   D = True   E = True

Although the most common cause of iron deficiency is reduced dietary intake, gastrointestinal blood loss may be causative, e.g. from oesophagitis, peptic ulcer, Crohn's disease and drinking cows' milk. Hookworm, not threadworm, infestation is a common cause worldwide. In thalassaemia major, the problem is excessive iron storage not deficiency.

56 A = False   B = True   C = True   D = True   E = False

After the first breath, pulmonary vascular resistance falls and pulmonary blood flow increases after the cord is clamped. Systemic vascular resistance increases. The increased pulmonary blood flow leads to an increase in pulmonary venous return, an increase in left atrial pressure and closure of the foramen ovale. Cardiac output increases after birth.

57 **A** = True   **B** = True   **C** = False   **D** = True   **E** = True

Lumbar puncture is hazardous in the presence of raised intracranial pressure, the signs of which include decreasing level of consciousness, papilloedema (often absent in young children), focal neurological signs and extensor plantar responses. A prolonged seizure also increases intracranial pressure. Lumbar puncture is also contraindicated in the presence of shock which may be present in meningococcaemia.

58 **A** = True   **B** = True   **C** = False   **D** = False   **E** = False

Transient proteinuria is common in normal children and may occur during acute febrile illness and after vigorous activity. However, urine should always be re-tested to ensure that proteinuria is not persistent. There is a poor correlation between proteinuria and urinary tract infection.

59 **A** = False   **B** = True   **C** = True   **D** = False   **E** = False

Nocturnal enuresis is common, affecting 10–15% of 5 year olds. There is an annual spontaneous remission rate of about 15% per year. Stress is usually a result and not the cause of enuresis. A family history is common. Only about 10% have a history of mild daytime wetting. The urine should always be checked using test strips and sent for culture. However, ultrasound is indicated only if a diagnosis of urinary infection is made.

60 **A** = False   **B** = True   **C** = False   **D** = True   **E** = True

In contrast to complex partial seizures, consciousness is usually retained in simple partial seizures. Breath-holding attacks follow an insult and a period of crying after which cyanosis and loss of consciousness ensue. In benign paroxysmal vertigo which occurs in children 1 to 5 years of age, the child experiences acute ataxia associated with vertigo and becomes frightened, unsteady and may fall, but consciousness is maintained. Hyperventilation is sometimes accompanied by loss of consciousness, probably as a result of hypocapnia and cerebral ischaemia. Children with Fallot's tetralogy experience episodes of severe cyanosis which may occasionally end in unconsciousness.

TEST 4
Answers to Multiple-Choice Questions

1 **A** = False **B** = True **C** = False **D** = True **E** = False

Health visitors are involved with children's care usually up to the age of 5 years. They play a central role in child health surveillance, and are particularly involved with children at risk of abuse or those with special needs. They usually take over the care from the midwife at 10 days after birth.

2 **A** = False **B** = False **C** = False **D** = False **E** = False

Health promotion may be carried out at individual, organisational, district, regional, or national level. Often local health promotion is more effective and responsive to local needs. Health promotion may involve disease prevention, health education and health protection by legislation or better design. The goals of health education are not achieved simply because the population acquires increased knowledge about health. There must be accompanying changes in behaviour. For example, health promotion programmes which increase knowledge of the harmful effects of cigarette smoking do not achieve their purposes until the prevalence of smoking decreases. It is generally agreed that exaggerating the harmful effects of certain behaviour is less effective than balanced discussion of the issues. The effect of health promotion often takes some time before it takes effect. For example, the effect of a stop smoking campaign may take some time before the prevalence of smoking reduces, which in turn takes time before the prevalence of coronary heart disease decreases.

3 **A** = True **B** = False **C** = False **D** = True **E** = False

Childminding is suitable for children up to the age of 8 years. All childminders need to register with the social services department. There are no compulsory statutory qualifications or training required for childminders at present. Generally speaking, the recommended childminder to child ratio is 1:3 for children under 5 and 1:6 for children over 5.

4 **A** = True **B** = False **C** = True **D** = True **E** = True

The Children Act 1989 introduced the key concept that the welfare of the child is paramount; the concept of parental responsibility rather than parental rights; and the concept that any delay in determining a question in relation to the upbringing of a child may prejudice his or her welfare. It has also replaced 'Place of Safety Order' with 'Emergency Protection Order'. The order lasts for 8 days, and can be renewed for a further 7 days.

5 A = True   **B** = True   **C** = True   **D** = False   **E** = False

Immunisation against *Haemophilus influenzae* Type B infection, fluoridation of water supplies, and using child-proof medicine containers attempt to prevent the onset of the conditions concerned in the first place, and are examples of primary prevention. The free-field distraction test aims to detect hearing loss in infants, and is an example of secondary prevention. Use of a steroid inhaler for an asthmatic child is an example of tertiary prevention.

6 A = True   **B** = False   **C** = True   **D** = True   **E** = True

The school entrant review usually takes place at about 5 years of age. All children should be seen by the school nurse for height and weight measurements, general developmental screening, visual acuity measurement by the Snellen chart, and hearing 'sweep' screening test. This is also an opportunity to establish a good relationship with the child's parents. Although all children used to be examined by the school doctor in the past, this has been found to be unnecessary. The current consensus is that the school doctor needs only to see selected students with identified problems.

7 A = False   **B** = False   **C** = False   **D** = True   **E** = True

Vaccines against rubella and polio are live. Meningococcus Type C vaccine is a killed vaccine, and diphtheria and tetanus vaccines contain toxoids.

8 A = True   **B** = False   **C** = False   **D** = True   **E** = True

Rubella vaccine is a live vaccine and is contraindicated in pregnancy. However, as there have been no documented cases of congenital rubella syndrome following accidental immunisation, termination of pregnancy should not be performed for accidental immunisation. Rubella vaccine is the main tool in eliminating congenital rubella syndrome, and universal immunisation between 1 and 18 months of age was introduced in 1988 in an attempt to establish herd immunity in the population. However, rubella immunisation at 11–13 years needs to be continued until those who were immunised in 1988 reach the age of 13 (i.e. about the year 2000). Rash, lymphadenopathy, arthritis and arthropathy, which are symptoms of rubella may occur in milder form after vaccination.

9 A = False   **B** = True   **C** = True   **D** = False   **E** = True

Breast or bottle milk can be appropriately given for a period after weaning. Chopped meat is suitable for most children after the age of 12 months. Sweetened drinks are not advisable for children as they encourage dental decay. Doorstep cows' milk is generally less suitable for infants, as it is high in protein and sodium content, and infants may be more liable to develop gastroenteritis. The high phosphate content of doorstep milk is also undesirable. In the past, the high phosphate content of unmodified cows' milk formulae used to cause hypocalcaemia.

10 A = False   **B** = True   **C** = False   **D** = True   **E** = True

Adolescents with constitutional growth delay often have a positive family history, and usually have pubertal delay. They may have short stature in childhood, which becomes more obvious at puberty when their classmates are rapidly growing. The delay in bone age and puberty are often similar. No treatment is usually required, and children often achieve normal adult height. Testosterone may be considered for some boys.

11 A = True   **B** = False   **C** = False   **D** = False   **E** = False

Thelarche is isolated early breast development without evidence of early puberty. This is quite common, and does not require investigation although follow up is required to ensure that this is not part of precocious puberty.

12 A = False   **B** = True   **C** = False   **D** = False   **E** = False

Childhood accident is the most common cause of mortality above the age of 1 year. Road traffic accidents represent about 2% of all accidents, but represent about 50% of all fatal accidents. Fire and drowning are the next most common causes of fatal accidents. Prevention of accidents may be achieved by education of parents and children, designs such as fire guards and child-proof medicine bottles, and legislation relating to seat-belts and vehicle safety.

13 A = True   **B** = False   **C** = True   **D** = True   **E** = True

Children at risk of deafness include those with a complicated neonatal history (e.g. low birth weight, birth asphyxia, severe unconjugated jaundice), a family history of deafness, cleft palate or abnormalities of the outer ear, recurrent otitis media, a history of meningitis, significantly delayed speech and syndromes such as first arch syndromes.

14 A = True   **B** = False   **C** = False   **D** = False   **E** = True

In bacterial meningitis, the CSF is usually turbid, with raised protein (greater than about 0.4 g/L), a low CSF glucose (CSF: blood glucose of 0.5 or less), and a predominance of neutrophils. Microscopy may show bacteria (coccobacilli may represent *Haemophilus influenzae*), and organisms are grown on culture.

  In viral meningitis, the CSF is usually clear with normal or slightly elevated protein and normal glucose levels. There is often an excess of lymphocytes. In TB meningitis, the protein level is raised and the glucose level is decreased.

15 A = False   **B** = True   **C** = True   **D** = False   **E** = True

Measles and rubella usually present with a maculopapular rash. Drug reaction also presents with a macular rash. Meningococcal septicaemia presents with a purpuric rash, and food allergy may present with an urticarial rash.

16 A = False   **B** = True   **C** = True   **D** = True   **E** = False

Although the incidence of tuberculosis has declined dramatically in the last century, it remains a problem in the immigrant population. Recently there has been an increase in the incidence of tuberculosis in countries where AIDS is endemic. The initial infection is either asymptomatic or presents with non-specific symptoms of fever or tiredness. The primary focus in the lung is often small and not visible on the chest X-ray. Regional lymph nodes are often enlarged. The risk for the development of meningitis is highest within a year of acquiring the primary infection.

17 **A** = True   **B** = False   **C** = True   **D** = True   **E** = False

Achondroplasia, neurofibromatosis and tuberous sclerosis are autosomal dominant. Albinism is autosomal recessive, and Duchenne muscular dystrophy is sex-linked recessive.

18 **A** = True   **B** = True   **C** = True   **D** = False   **E** = False

Most full-term babies pass meconium within 24 hours after birth, and failure to do so should be investigated. However, preterm babies often fail to pass meconium within the first day without an organic cause. Important organic causes include anal stenosis or atresia, Hirschsprung disease, cystic fibrosis and hypothyroidism.

19 **A** = False   **B** = True   **C** = True   **D** = True   **E** = False

Breast-feeding has many advantages. These include an appropriate intake of nutrients including proteins, fats and electrolytes. The risks of infection (especially gastrointestinal) and atopy are reduced. Although there is less risk with breast-feeding, cows' milk intolerance is possible in breast-feeding, as cows' milk protein ingested by the mother can be secreted in her milk. Breast-feeding may cause jaundice, although it is almost always harmless.

20 **A** = False   **B** = False   **C** = True   **D** = False   **E** = True

Boys with Klinefelter's syndrome have the XXY karyotype. The incidence is about 1 in 1000 liveborn males. They characteristically have tall stature, gynaecomastia, poorly developed secondary sexual characteristics, and small testes. They have reduced fertility.

21 **A** = True   **B** = False   **C** = False   **D** = True   **E** = False

The causes of vomiting in the first week of life are infections, metabolic disorders (e.g. galactosaemia), and congenital abnormalities of the gut such as duodenal or jejunal atresia. Pyloric stenosis usually does not present until 3 weeks after birth. Coeliac disease usually presents after 3 months of age. Appendicitis is rare in infancy.

22 **A** = True   **B** = True   **C** = True   **D** = True   **E** = True

Clinical features of cystic fibrosis include failure to thrive, pancreatic insufficiency, chest infections and bronchiectasis, meconium ileus, rectal prolapse, intussusception, and obstructive liver disease.

23 **A** = True   **B** = True   **C** = True   **D** = True   **E** = True

Non-organic failure to thrive may be due to social factors such as poor housing, unemployment, single parent, marital discord, or to maternal problems such as mental illness, drug or alcohol abuse. It can also be due to poor parental knowledge about feeding requirements and techniques.

24 **A** = True　　**B** = True　　**C** = True　　**D** = True　　**E** = True

There are many factors which may precipitate an attack of asthma. These include infection (especially rhinovirus and para-influenza), allergens (especially pollen), exercise, emotional disturbance, and physical irritation (e.g. cold air).

25 **A** = True　　**B** = True　　**C** = False　　**D** = True　　**E** = False

Physical signs which would indicate that an asthmatic attack in a child is severe include the inability to speak, eat or drink, cyanosis, tachycardia, pulsus paradox of 20 mmHg or more, use of accessory muscles of respiration, intercostal and subcostal recession, and tachypnoea. The loudness of wheezing is not a good indicator of the severity of the attack. A silent chest indicates that the airway obstruction is extremely severe, and there is little air moving in and out of the chest.

26 **A** = True　　**B** = True　　**C** = False　　**D** = False　　**E** = True

Acute otitis media is often preceded by a viral upper respiratory tract infection. Temporary hearing loss is common. Severe otitis media rarely spreads causing mastoiditis and meningitis. As *Haemophilus influenzae* is often responsible, benzylpenicillin is not the optimal treatment. Amoxycillin, erythromycin or a cephalosporin would be more appropriate. Decongestants have not been proven to be beneficial.

27 **A** = True　　**B** = True　　**C** = True　　**D** = True　　**E** = True

Pneumonia in infants and children can be caused by a wide variety of organisms. *Pneumococcus* is the most common bacterial cause. *Haemophilus influenzae* pneumonia may accompany either otitis media or epiglottitis. *Chylamydia* may be acquired during delivery, and cause conjunctivitis and pneumonia in early infancy. *Mycoplasma pneumoniae* affects mainly older children.

28 **A** = False　　**B** = False　　**C** = False　　**D** = False　　**E** = False

Cyanosis appears when there is more than about 5 g reduced haemoglobbin/100 ml and is therefore more difficult to detect in the presence of anaemia. Finger clubbing is due to arterial oxygen desaturation, but does not occur until late in the first year. Administration of 100% oxygen can distinguish between cardiovascular and respiratory causes of cyanosis in infants. Oxygen saturation increases much more in infants with respiratory disease than those with cyanotic heart disease. In transposition of the great arteries, cyanosis may not be apparent at birth because the patent ductus arteriosus allows mixing of the two circulations.

29 **A** = False　　**B** = True　　**C** = False　　**D** = False　　**E** = True

Atrial septal defects are usually asymptomatic, as the left to right shunt is small, although rarely large defects may cause cardiac failure in childhood. Symptoms do not usually occur until the third decade or later. As the difference in pressure between the two atria is small, the risk of bacterial endocarditis is extremely small or non-existent. The characteristic signs are an ejection systolic murmur loudest at the left upper sternal edge, and wide fixed splitting of the second heart sound. The murmur is **not** due to shunting of blood across the atria, but is due to high blood flow across the pulmonary valve.

30 A = True   **B** = True   **C** = True   **D** = True   **E** = True

Hypercyanotic attacks associated with Fallot's tetralogy are due to an increase in the right ventricular tract obstruction and the right to left shunt. They occur especially in the morning or following excessive crying or exertion. The child becomes increasingly cyanosed, and may lose consciousness. During the attack, the murmur may disappear or decrease in intensity. Although rarely fatal, these attacks can cause convulsions and brain damage. The child should be placed in the knee–elbow position in 100% oxygen. This may help to reduce the return of venous blood from the lower limbs to the heart, similar to the squatting position which is often adopted. Propranolol may be used to treat or prevent attacks by relieving infundibular spasm.

31 A = True   **B** = True   **C** = False   **D** = False   **E** = False

Febrile convulsions are most common during viral infections, especially upper respiratory tract infection. Pertussis and MMR immunisations may be followed by febrile convulsions, especially in those with a past history. Most febrile convulsions are of the tonic-clonic type. The child may go limp, lose consciousness, and there may be generalised jerks. About 10% of febrile convulsions are unilateral. Most febrile convulsions last less than 10 minutes. More serious pathology especially meningitis should be considered in longer convulsions. In fact, the possibility of meningitis should always be considered and if any doubt exists, a lumbar puncture is indicated.

32 A = True   **B** = True   **C** = True   **D** = True   **E** = False

Sodium valproate is effective in the treatment of absence seizures (primary generalised epilepsy) and generalised tonic-clonic seizures, but less effective in the treatment of complex partial seizures. The most common side-effects, nausea and vomiting, may be minimised by giving the drug after meals. Other side-effects include obesity due to increased appetite and reversible alopecia. It can rarely cause fatal hepatic toxicity, which occurs in the early stages of treatment. Hence, it is prudent to check liver function tests before treatment.

33 A = False   **B** = True   **C** = True   **D** = True   **E** = True

Children with Duchenne muscular dystrophy show myopathic but non-specific EMG abnormalities. Muscle biopsy is used to make a definitive diagnosis. Chorionic villous biopsy followed by DNA testing can be used to make an antenatal diagnosis. Children with Duchenne muscular dystrophy develop scoliosis, resulting in chest deformity. Death in the late teens or early twenties results from cardiomyopathy, pneumonia or respiratory failure.

34 A = False   **B** = False   **C** = True   **D** = True   **E** = False

Children with infantile autism present before 2½ years of age. The characteristic features are lack of responsiveness to other people, gross deficits in language development, and rituals which the child is extremely resistant to change. There may be stereotyped movements and inappropriate attachment to objects. There may be echolalia (repetition of what other people say) or echopraxia (repetition of what others do). However, there are no hallucinations, delusions or loosening of associations which are characteristic of childhood schizophrenia.

35 A = True   **B** = True   **C** = True   **D** = True   **E** = True

Acute leukaemia may present in many ways. There may be non-specific symptoms such as general malaise, lethargy or anorexia. Presenting symptoms may be due to a fall in haemoglobin (anaemia), white cell count (unusually severe and frequent infections), or platelets (easy bruising or haemorrhages). It may also present with bone and joint pain due to leukaemic infiltration.

36 A = False   **B** = False   **C** = True   **D** = False   **E** = True

Trimethoprim is often the best first-line treatment of a urinary tract infection. Many *E. coli* infections are resistant to amoxycillin. Co-trimoxazole contains trimethoprim and sulphamethoxazole, and has more side-effects than trimethoprim alone. Failure to respond clinically within 48 hours generally means that the organism is resistant to the antibiotic, and it should be changed accordingly, depending on culture and sensitivity. Trimethoprim and nitrofurantoin are suitable prophylactic agents in children with significant vesico-ureteric reflux, as they are excreted in the urine in high concentrations. They should be given at night, as this will allow the drug to act for a longer time before voiding.

37 A = True   **B** = False   **C** = True   **D** = False   **E** = True

Precocious puberty may be due to gonadotrophin-dependent causes. It may be constitutional, especially in girls or due to lesions of the hypothalamic–pituitary region such as tumours. Boys have a much higher incidence of the latter. Gonadotrophin-independent causes include ovarian or testicular tumours and adrenal hyperplasia or tumours. Turner syndrome causes absent puberty and primary amenorrhoea.

38 A = True   **B** = True   **C** = False   **D** = True   **E** = False

Vitamin D is manufactured by two sources in the body. The first source is from the conversion of 7-dehydrocholesterol to vitamin D3 in the skin on exposure to the sun's ultraviolet radiation. The second source is ingested vitamin D. In both cases, vitamin D is converted to 25-hydroxycholecalciferol in the liver, followed by conversion to 1,25-hydroxycholecalciferol in the kidney. Childhood rickets may be due to a vitamin deficiency (e.g. caused by dietary deficiency, malabsorption or lack of sunshine) or low phosphate (e.g. due to renal loss of phosphate in renal tubular acidosis), or chronic renal failure.

39 **A** = False   **B** = True   **C** = True   **D** = True   **E** = True

Meningitis, especially if caused by *Haemophilus influenzae*, may be complicated by sensori-neural deafness, hydrocephalus and subdural collection of fluid. Subdural collection of fluid is especially common in infants, and may cause pyrexia, vomiting and bulging fontanelle which may resemble recurrence of the meningitis. Other neurological complications include epilepsy, cerebral palsy and cranial nerve palsies.

40 **A** = False   **B** = True   **C** = True   **D** = False   **E** = True

Erythema infectiosum, also known as fifth disease or 'slapped cheek' disease, is caused by a parvovirus. Children present with a rash initially on the cheeks with sparing around the mouth, giving rise to the 'slapped cheek' appearance, and fever. The rash spreads to the trunk and limbs after about 2–3 days and may be pruritic. Cervical lymphanopathy may occur. Asymmetrical arthritis may develop a few days after the rash. Infection during pregnancy may result in stillbirth.

41 **A** = True   **B** = True   **C** = True   **D** = True   **E** = True

Anorexia nervosa mainly affects women in their late teens or early twenties. Fear of obesity while underweight, distortion of body image (believing that she is much fatter than she actually is) are characteristic. Evidence of hormonal disturbance such as amenorrhoea is often present. About 5% of cases occur in men. Anorexia nervosa may be associated with laxative abuse or induced vomiting which may cause hypokalaemia. Psychological treatment includes cognitive behavioural therapy, individual therapy, family therapy or a combination of these. Patients may require in-patient treatment for bedrest or naso-gastric feeding if the condition is severe.

42 **A** = False   **B** = True   **C** = False   **D** = True   **E** = False

Breath-holding attacks affect children aged between 6 months and 5 years. They usually follow minor trauma, emotional upset or a tantrum. The child often cries, then appears to hold his or her breath, and becomes cyanosed. The child may lose consciousness, and may even have a few jerks. However, recovery is rapid. These attacks are harmless and self-limiting, and require no treatment other than reassurance for the parents.

43 **A** = False   **B** = False   **C** = True   **D** = True   **E** = True

About 80% of diaphragmatic hernias occur on the left side through the foramen of Bochdalek. Hernias of the foramen of Morgagni rarely cause symptoms in the neonatal period. Diagnosis is sometimes made on antenatal ultrasound. Lung hypoplasia and persistent foetal circulation are major contributors to morbidity and mortality.

44 A = False   **B** = True   **C** = True   **D** = False   **E** = False

Von Willebrand's disease, which is inherited as an autosomal dominant trait, is the most common inherited bleeding disorder. It can be asymptomatic, and diagnosis often follows a positive family history. Common symptoms include epistaxis, prolonged oozing from wounds, post-operative bleeding and menorrhagia. The last symptom is often the most troublesome. The normal neonate tends to have increased levels of Von Willebrand factor which makes the diagnosis difficult in the neonatal period.

45 A = True   **B** = False   **C** = False   **D** = False   **E** = True

Recurrent abdominal pain is common, affecting 10% of the school age population. In the vast majority of cases, the pain is periumbilical or epigastric. Pain further from the midline is more likely to have an organic aetiology which is present in 10% or less of cases. Pain occurring at mealtimes is more likely to be attention seeking than due to food allergy. Recurrent abdominal pain is often associated with pallor, headache and vomiting.

46 A = True   **B** = True   **C** = True   **D** = False   **E** = True

Parental smoking significantly increases the incidence of pneumonia and wheezing in infancy but does not seem to cause a significant increase in asthma admissions. Maternal smoking during pregnancy significantly increases the risk of sudden infant death syndrome. After birth the risk is higher if both parents smoke than if one parent smokes, indicating that exposure to smoke after birth is also a risk factor.

47 A = True   **B** = False   **C** = True   **D** = True   **E** = True

Whilst sodium valproate causes mild hair loss in some patients, phenytoin may cause hirsutism. Phenytoin is used less often nowadays due to its potential toxicity. Hair pulling, which may be a habit or indicate more serious psychological problems, is associated with partial alopecia. Traction alopecia may occur in young girls who have tight ponytails.

48 A = True   **B** = False   **C** = True   **D** = False   **E** = False

Pneumonia (especially if the upper lobes are involved) and tonsillitis may cause neck stiffness. Headache with neck stiffness is very unlikely to be caused by migraine and meningitis should be excluded.

49 A = False   **B** = False   **C** = True   **D** = True   **E** = True

Cardiac failure in infants is often caused by a large left to right shunt. Fallot's tetralogy is characterised by cyanosis and not cardiac failure. The cardinal signs of cardiac failure are tachycardia, tachypnoea and hepatomegaly. Sweating, especially during feeding, vomiting and poor weight gain also occur.

50 A = False   **B** = False   **C** = True   **D** = False   **E** = True

Signs or symptoms of narcotic withdrawal occur at about 24 hours and include irritability, tremor, hypertonicity, vomiting and convulsions. Hyaline membrane disease is uncommon because heroin stimulates surfactant production. Nalo-xone may precipitate acute withdrawal and should not be given. Graded doses of morphine are used to control symptoms, which may persist for several weeks. These babies have a significantly increased risk of sudden infant death syndrome.

51 A = False   B = True   C = False   D = True   E = True

Most cases of acute viral laryngotracheitis are caused by parainfluenza virus but epiglottitis is caused by *Haemophilus influenzae* Type B. This is a severe life-threatening illness accompanied by septicaemia, severe upper airway obstruction, drooling and difficulty in swallowing. Elective endotracheal intubation by a skilled anaesthetist should be carried out once the condition is suspected. No attempt should be made to visualise the throat beforehand as this may precipitate respiratory arrest.

52 A = True   B = True   C = False   D = True   E = True

Hypoglycaemia especially if accompanied by small genitalia in boys may indicate growth hormone deficiency. Causes of hypoglycaemia also include other hormone deficiencies (e.g. glucocorticoids), enzyme deficiencies (e.g. galactosaemia), glycogen storage disease, liver disease, alcohol, hyperinsulinism and fatty acid oxidation defects (e.g. MCAD deficiency).

53 A = True   B = False   C = True   D = True   E = False

Transient painful swollen joints are common in Henoch–Schönlein purpura in addition to the characteristic rash, abdominal pain and renal involvement. Idiopathic thrombocytopenic purpura causes cutaneous and mucosal but not joint bleeding. Bone pain and arthralgia are common in the child presenting with acute lymphatic leukaemia. The 'hand–foot syndrome' resulting from symmetrical infarction of the metacarpals and metatarsals is common in infants with sickle-cell disease while painful crises involving joints usually begin after the age of 3 or 4 years.

54 A = True   B = False   C = True   D = True   E = True

In Perthes' disease, the proximal femoral epiphysis becomes avascular and dies. The condition affects children aged 3 to 10 years, and is more common in boys. Perthes' disease most often presents with a limp whereas slipped upper femoral epiphysis which affects older children usually presents with pain.

55 A = True   B = False   C = True   D = False   E = False

Christmas disease, like haemophilia A, has X-linked inheritance. Ataxia telangiectasia is inherited as an autosomal recessive disorder. Pierre Robin syndrome is not an inherited condition.

56 A = False   B = False   C = True   D = True   E = False

Neuroblastoma, the second most common solid tumour after brain tumour, may present with constitutional symptoms, an abdominal mass, a mass in the neck, or symptoms due to compression of other structures. Many children have metastases at presentation and the prognosis is much worse than that of Wilms' tumour.

57 A = False   **B** = False   **C** = False   **D** = True   **E** = True

Chickenpox, caused by a DNA virus, varicella zoster, usually has no prodromal symptoms. The incubation period is usually about 14 days (11 to 21 days). Chickenpox in pregnancy can cause intrauterine growth retardation, eye abnormalities and serious neurodevelopmental problems in offspring. Secondary skin infection is the most common complication but neurological problems such as aseptic meningitis, encephalitis, Guillain–Barré syndrome, transverse myelitis and acute cerebellaritis can occur.

58 A = True   **B** = True   **C** = True   **D** = True   **E** = True

Most children who wheeze either have wheezy bronchitis, viral bronchiolitis or asthma, but is important to consider other causes particularly cystic fibrosis and gastro-oesophageal reflux. Enlarged nodes in tuberculosis, vascular ring, mediastinal cysts and tumours may compress airways. One should always consider foreign bodies particularly if wheeze is unilateral.

59 A = False   **B** = True   **C** = False   **D** = True   **E** = False

Severe learning difficulty is more common in boys, partly due to inherited conditions such as the fragile X syndrome. Behavioural problems are common. Mild to moderate learning difficulties are more common in boys with Duchenne muscular dystrophy. Girls with Turner's syndrome usually have normal intelligence.

60 A = False   **B** = False   **C** = True   **D** = False   **E** = False

Vesicoureteric reflux is found in about 40% of children with a urinary tract infection. Its importance lies in its association with renal scarring which occurs in about one-third of children with reflux. Mild reflux may occur after bladder infection, hence it is best to defer investigation of reflux for a few weeks after a urinary tract infection. Vesicoureteric reflux is best demonstrated by micturating cystogram, although isotope studies may be acceptable in older children who can cooperate with a request to micturate.

TEST 5
Answers to Multiple-Choice Questions

1 **A** = True **B** = False **C** = False **D** = False **E** = False

The 1944 Education Act states that parents must ensure that their children of compulsory school age (between 5 to 16 years) receive education suited to them. Although the vast majority of children receive their education by regular attendance at school, this need not be so. For example, they may receive their education at home. However, local education authorities have a duty to provide free schooling at the statutory school age. Although many local education authorities provide nursery education for some children between 3 and 5 years old, this is not statutory. Children attend primary school between the ages of 5 and 11 years, and secondary school between the ages of 11 and 16 years. Beyond the age of 16, there is a choice between sixth-form colleges, sixth forms, or colleges of further education.

2 **A** = False **B** = False **C** = False **D** = False **E** = True

Health education is now firmly established as part of the National Curriculum, and has been defined comprehensively. It includes psychological aspects, substance misuse, family-life education, sex education, safety, health-related exercise, personal hygiene and environmental aspects. Teachers are encouraged to develop health education as cross-curricular themes, to be integrated with other subjects rather than as a separate subject, so that all teachers may be involved in health education.

3 **A** = False **B** = True **C** = True **D** = False **E** = True

The spirit of the 1989 Children Act is that children should remain with their families whenever possible. Hence, the number of children under the care of local authorities has decreased, and the use of residential homes has been reduced in favour of foster care. It was found that deprived children (e.g. those whose families receive income support) have a higher chance of being in care. Black children have a higher chance, and Asian children have a lower chance of being in care.

4 **A** = False **B** = True **C** = True **D** = False **E** = False

An education supervision order can be made on a child of compulsory school age. It is usually made only if the school attendance is unsatisfactory. While it places the child under the supervision of a local education authority, it does not exclude either the parents or the child from participating in making further decisions relating to his or her further education. The order lasts initially for 1 year.

5   A = False   **B** = False   **C** = True   **D** = True   **E** = True

There are a few important principles for child health surveillance. Firstly, history and observation of the child rather than screening tests are the most important tools. Secondly, parents and different health professionals should cooperate to make child health surveillance a success. In general, the health visitor and the school nurse are the central professionals in the delivery of child health surveillance to pre-school and school-aged children.

6   A = True   **B** = False   **C** = True   **D** = False   **E** = False

Colour vision defects are usually X-linked recessive conditions, and are therefore much more common in boys than in girls. There are no treatments. However, as they are barriers for entrance into some professions, detection while at school allows suitable career guidance. The most commonly used screening test is the Ishihara test, where the subject has to identify a number from a constellation of colour dots. This is a very sensitive test and detects most colour vision defects, including minor ones. However, it is unsuitable for career guidance as it gives no information on the severity or which colours are being confused. The City University Plates are more suitable for detailed career guidance.

7   A = True   **B** = False   **C** = False   **D** = True   **E** = True

Oral polio vaccine, combined diphtheria, pertussis and tetanus vaccines, and *Haemophilus influenzae* Type B are usually given in three doses between 2 and 4 months of age. Combined measles, mumps and rubella (MMR) vaccine is usually given between the age of 12 and 18 months. A new regime where a second dose of MMR is administered just before school entry is being introduced.

8   A = False   **B** = True   **C** = False   **D** = False   **E** = False

Whooping cough may be caused by either *Bordetella pertussis* or less commonly *Bordetella parapertussis*. It has the worst prognosis in infancy. The risk of developing the disease is reduced by about 90%, and the child usually has milder disease even if he or she develops the illness following immunisation. Whooping cough has an incubation period of 1 to 2 weeks, a catarrhal phase of 1 to 2 weeks, and a paroxysmal phase which may last a few weeks. The child may have a residual cough for weeks to months.

9   A = False   **B** = True   **C** = True   **D** = True   **E** = False

Cow's milk intolerance is often over-diagnosed due to the large number of symptoms attributed to it. It can occur in totally breast-fed infants, as cows' milk protein ingested by the mother may be excreted in breast-milk. It is an uncommon cause of wheeze in infancy, but can be associated with occult blood loss causing anaemia. Children with true milk intolerance may be given either soya formulae or hydroxylated protein formulae. The symptoms usually improve as the child gets older.

10 A = False **B** = True **C** = True **D** = True **E** = True

Turner's syndrome affects about 1 in 2500 liveborn girls. The karyotype can be either XO or a mosaic XX/XO. The characteristic features include short stature, short webbed neck, increased carrying angle at the elbow and widely-spaced nipples, although short stature may be present with minimal other clinical features. There are either no ovaries or streak ovaries only, and girls may present with primary amenorrhoea. It may be associated with coarctation of the aorta. Although affected girls are not usually growth hormone deficient, treatment with high-dose human growth hormone can increase final adult height.

11 A = True **B** = True **C** = False **D** = True **E** = False

Primitive reflexes such as the Moro reflex, stepping reflex, grasp reflex and the asymmetric tonic neck reflex should disappear before 6 months of age. Persistence beyond this time should arouse concern. The Moro reflex is consistently present in newborns and disappears before the age of 6 months. An asymmetrical Moro reflex should arouse suspicion of a local cause such as a fracture or neurological abnormality. The parachute reaction, in which the child extends the arms if rapidly lowered when held in the ventral position, is abnormal if absent.

12 A = True **B** = True **C** = True **D** = True **E** = True

The reduction in numbers of childhood accidents is one of the key targets in the 'Health of the Nation', with the target of reduction by at least one-third by the year 2005. Childhood accidents increase with lower social class. Boys have twice the rate of accidental head injury than girls. Prevention can take place at an individual level (e.g. in general practice consultation), at an organisational level (e.g. in schools or hospitals), or at national or international level. Education, good designs, and legislation are all important methods of preventing childhood accidents.

13 A = True **B** = False **C** = True **D** = True **E** = False

Separation anxiety disorder is characterised by a fear of separation from a major attachment figure as the main focus of anxiety. It usually develops from an early age. Excessive fear of dogs may be due to animal phobia. Stranger anxiety is a normal development from the age of 9 months to 1 year. If it is severe, it may be classified as social anxiety disorder of childhood.

14 A = True **B** = True **C** = True **D** = True **E** = False

Sudden infant death syndrome has an incidence of just under 1:1000 live births, with a peak incidence at between 2 and 3 months after birth and in the winter months. Risk factors include prematurity, low birth weight, male sex, higher order births, parental low social group and parental smoking. It has also been shown that babies nursed supine have a lower incidence than those nursed prone.

15 A = True   **B** = True   **C** = False   **D** = False   **E** = False

Chickenpox may cause ataxia due to post-infectious cerebellaritis. Pneumonia occurs especially in children with immunodeficiency. Subacute sclerosing panen-cephalitis and Koplik's spots are both features of measles. Cold sores are due to herpes simplex infection.

16 A = True   **B** = False   **C** = False   **D** = False   **E** = False

The Mantoux test is given intradermally in the upper third of the flexor surface of the forearm. Usually, 0.1 ml containing 1 tuberculin unit is given. A control may be given in the other forearm. The test should be read between 48 and 72 hours, and the result is indicated by the area of induration rather than the area of erythema.

17 A = True   **B** = True   **C** = False   **D** = False   **E** = True

G6PD deficiency, haemophilia A and B, and chronic granulomatous disease are sex-linked recessive disorders. Galactosaemia is autosomal recessive, and congenital spherocytosis is autosomal dominant.

18 A = False   **B** = True   **C** = True   **D** = False   **E** = False

Haemolysis is the major cause of jaundice in the first 24 hours of life. This is the most dangerous form of jaundice, as unconjugated hyperbilirubinaemia can increase rapidly and cause kernicterus. Rhesus disease used to be the most important cause, but with routine administration of anti-D after delivery in rhesus negative women, ABO incompatibility is now more common. Non-immune haemolysis can be due to glucose 6-phosphate dehydrogenase (G6PD) deficiency or to congenital spherocytosis. Other causes of neonatal jaundice in the first 24 hours include sepsis and congenital infection.

19 A = True   **B** = False   **C** = True   **D** = True   **E** = True

Motor tics are repeated, involuntary, purposeless and rapid movements. Vocal tics are sudden utterances which serve no apparent purpose. There is a continuous spectrum of tic disorders, ranging from transient simple tics to complex multiple incapacitating tics as in de la Tourette's syndrome. About 10% of children may have experienced transient tics, but Tourette's syndrome is very rare. Motor tics may consist of shoulder shrugging, neck jerking or eye blinking. Vocal tics may consist of hissing, throat clearing, repeating certain words, or even repeating obscene words (coprolalia).

20 A = True   **B** = True   **C** = False   **D** = False   **E** = False

An average 9-month old child can sit steadily for a few minutes and stand holding on to furniture. He or she can creep forward in the prone position, but cannot creep upstairs until about 15 months. The child can click two bricks together by imitation, but cannot build a tower of two cubes until he or she is 15 months of age. The child can understand a few words, and babble, but cannot say two or three words with meaning until after 1 year of age.

21 **A** = True   **B** = True   **C** = False   **D** = False   **E** = True

Congenital hypertrophic pyloric stenosis is more common in males than in females, and there is often a positive family history. It usually develops between 3 and 7 weeks after birth. A pyloric mass can be felt with the examiner's left hand in the right hypochondrium when the baby is feeding. Ultrasound is now the best way to diagnose the condition if a pyloric mass cannot be palpated; it has replaced barium studies to a large extent.

22 **A** = True   **B** = True   **C** = True   **D** = True   **E** = False

Anal fissure is the most common cause of rectal bleeding in children. Other causes include gastrointestinal infection, inflammatory bowel disease (Crohn's disease or ulcerative colitis), and intestinal polyps. Rectal bleeding in intussusception (redcurrant jelly stool) follows bouts of screaming and pallor. Occult blood loss may occur in cows' milk intolerance.

23 **A** = False   **B** = True   **C** = True   **D** = False   **E** = False

Stridor is caused by the narrowing of the airway from the glottis to the trachea during inspiration. The most common cause in a child is acute laryngotracheitis (croup). Other less common causes include a foreign body, acute epiglottitis, or angiooedema. Asthma affects the bronchi and causes wheeze. Pneumonia and cystic fibrosis affect the lung parenchyma.

24 **A** = True   **B** = False   **C** = True   **D** = True   **E** = True

Drugs given by inhalation have a more direct and rapid action on the lungs than when administered orally. The systemic side-effects are also less frequent. Inhalers often deliver less than 5% of the drugs to the lower respiratory tract, and nebulisers usually deliver 10% or less of the drugs to the lower respiratory tract. The choice of drug depends on the pattern of the disease of the child. If there are daily symptoms with acute attacks, or long periods of reversible airway obstruction, then prophylactic drugs should be given.

25 **A** = False   **B** = False   **C** = False   **D** = False   **E** = False

If the initial symptoms are moderate or severe, systematic steroids should be given even if the child improves after nebulised salbutamol. The effect of salbutamol may wear off quickly. Usually, prednisolone 1–2 mg/kg/day is given for a period of 5 days. Oxygen can be given at a high concentration if necessary in contrast to older adults with obstructive airway disease. A chest X-ray is unnecessary unless clinical signs suggest pneumonia or pneumothorax.

26 **A** = True   **B** = False   **C** = False   **D** = True   **E** = True

Whooping cough is mainly caused by *Bordetella pertussis*, but *Bordetella parapertussis* and some viruses can cause illness resembling whooping cough. The catarrhal phase resembles an upper respiratory infection with cough and pyrexia. This is followed by the paroxysmal phase with bouts of paroxysmal cough, which may end with vomiting or a whoop. Pertussis in infants may be particularly severe with associated apnoea attacks. It is often associated with a high lymphocyte count in the early stage of the disease. *Bordetella pertussis* is often difficult to culture, and a perinasal swab from the nasopharynx should be taken for microbiological examination.

27   **A** = True   **B** = True   **C** = True   **D** = False   **E** = True

Foreign body inhalation in children is most common in boys in the younger age group. Nuts are the most common culprits. The foreign body is frequently lodged in the right main bronchus. Symptoms depend on the size of the foreign body and where it is lodged. The symptoms may be choking, cyanosis, cough, wheezing or stridor. If the foreign body causes complete obstruction in the upper airway, there is sudden onset of choking with cyanosis. If it is lodged lower down in a segment of the bronchus, collapse of the segment will occur.

28   **A** = True   **B** = False   **C** = True   **D** = False   **E** = True

Shunting of blood from the left to the right side of the heart can occur at the arterial level (patent ductus arteriosus, where blood flows from the aorta to the pulmonary artery); at the ventricular level (ventricular septal defect, where blood flows from the left ventricle to the right ventricle) or the atrial level (atrial septal defect, where blood flows from the left atrium to the right atrium).

29   **A** = True   **B** = True   **C** = True   **D** = False   **E** = True

Delayed closure of the ductus arteriosus is more common in premature babies. In infants, a large defect may cause cardiac failure. However, patent ductus arteriosus is often asymptomatic in the older child. The characteristic findings are bounding pulses with wide pulse pressure, and a continuous machinery murmur loudest at the left upper sternal edge or below the left clavicle, and radiating to the back. In the neonate, surgical closure may be necessary because of cardiac failure or persistent symptoms such as apnoea in babies recovering from idiopathic respiratory distress syndrome. In the older asymptomatic child, surgical closure should also be undertaken to prevent the risk of infective endocarditis.

30   **A** = False   **B** = True   **C** = True   **D** = True   **E** = True

Although hypertension is more likely to be secondary to other diseases in children than in adults, essential hypertension does occur in children and adolescents. Children with essential hypertension are more likely to be overweight and have a positive family history. Hypertension is usually asymptomatic in children, but if sustained or rising rapidly, can cause neurological symptoms and symptoms of cardiac failure. All children with hypertension should be investigated for underlying diseases. These include renal disease, coarctation of the aorta, endocrine diseases such as Cushing's disease or salt-retaining types of congenital adrenal hyperplasia, or phaeochromocytoma.

31 **A** = False   **B** = False   **C** = True   **D** = False   **E** = True

Absence attacks usually present when the child is between 3 and 10 years, and are more common in girls than in boys. Affected children often have a positive family history. The child often suddenly loses awareness, and looks vacant for a few seconds. The child recovers rapidly and resumes his or her previous activity. There is no loss of consciousness. An EEG typically shows a characteristic 3 cycles/second spike and wave pattern. Treatment is with either sodium valproate or ethosuximide.

32 **A** = True   **B** = False   **C** = True   **D** = True   **E** = True

Phenytoin is effective against both generalised tonic-clonic epilepsy and complex partial seizures. However, it is not effective against absence seizures. It is given twice daily. Phenytoin potentially interacts with many other drugs and has long-term neurological side-effects such as cerebellar ataxia and deterioration in intellectual functioning. Other side-effects include hirsuitism and gum hyperplasia. It is less often used today because of its side-effects.

33 **A** = False   **B** = False   **C** = False   **D** = True   **E** = True

Cerebral palsy may be defined as a non-progressive disorder of posture and movement due to a defect of or damage to the developing brain. Birth trauma is an uncommon cause and intrapartum asphyxia is now thought to be less important as an aetiological factor. The incidence is about 0.25% of all live births. Tuberous sclerosis is a progressive disorder. Kernicterus (choreoathetosis, epilepsy and deafness caused by hyperbilirubinaemia in the neonatal period) is a cause of cerebral palsy, but is becoming much less common with improved neonatal care.

34 **A** = True   **B** = False   **C** = True   **D** = True   **E** = True

Neurofibromatosis is a autosomal dominant disorder. There are two distinct types: peripheral neurofibromatosis (NF1) with childhood onset, and central neurofibromatosis (NF2) with onset in early adulthood. NF1 often presents with café-au-lait spots (at least 5 over 5 mm in prepubertal patients and at least 5 over 15 mm in post-pubertal patients). Patients may develop optic nerve glioma, astrocytomas, neurofibromas and meningiomas. Kyphoscoliosis and renal artery stenosis are recognised features. NF2 presents with bilateral acoustic neuromas which seldom become malignant. Adenoma sebaceum (facial angiofibromata) is a sign of tuberous sclerosis.

35 **A** = False   **B** = False   **C** = True   **D** = False   **E** = True

Idiopathic thrombocytopenic purpura is not an inherited disorder. It usually affects children between 2 and 5 years of age with excessive bruising or epistaxis. The child is otherwise well. A full blood count usually shows no other abnormalities apart from a low platelet count. An accompanying low neutrophil count should raise the possibility of acute leukaemia. The disease usually remits spontaneously within 2 months, and about three-quarters of cases remit within 6 months. Those at risk of severe haemorrhage can be treated with a course of prednisolone provided a bone marrow examination has been carried out to exclude acute leukaemia.

36 A = True   **B** = False   **C** = True   **D** = False   **E** = True

Vesico-ureteric reflux is usually congenital in origin. Its presence with urinary tract infection may lead to renal scarring, and therefore must be taken seriously. It may be demonstrated by micturating cystourethrogram (MCU) or by isotope studies. It is present in about one-third of children with a urinary tract infection. Reflux is graded from Grade I to Grade V according to the International Classification of Reflux. Grade I is defined to be reflux in the ureter only, while in Grade V, there is gross dilatation of ureter, renal pelvis and calyces.

37 A = True   **B** = True   **C** = True   **D** = True   **E** = False

Secondary amenorrhoea is defined as absence of menstruation for 6 months or more in a woman who previously had regular menstruation. The most common cause is pregnancy. Pathological causes may be at the hypothalamic level (e.g. weight loss, stress); pituitary level (e.g. pituitary tumour), ovarian level (e.g. polycystic ovarian syndrome, premature ovarian failure) or uterine level (recent hysterectomy, Asherman's syndrome). While most children with Turner's syndrome have primary amenorrhoea, some (especially those with mosaic Turner's syndrome) have a few scanty periods before they stop.

38 A = True   **B** = True   **C** = True   **D** = True   **E** = False

Congenital adrenal hyperplasia is an autosomal recessive disorder caused by deficiency of one of the five enzymes responsible required for the synthesis of cortisol. The signs depend on which enzyme is deficient. The most common form is 21-hydroxylase deficiency in which androgen excess results in ambiguous genitalia in the female. In the salt-losing forms of 21-hydroxylase deficiency, aldosterone deficiency leads to excess renal sodium loss, causing vomiting, poor feeding, dehydration, hyponatraemia and hyperkalaemia at the end of the first week. Mild cases may present later with hirsuitism and delayed menarche. 11-beta-hydroxylase deficiency results in increased deoxycorticosterone which has salt-retaining properties, causing hypertension.

39 A = False   **B** = False   **C** = True   **D** = False   **E** = True

The most common organisms causing gastroenteritis in children are rotaviruses which mainly affect children under 18 months of age. Rotavirus infection can be particularly severe in young infants. Children who are breast-fed are less likely to develop gastroenteritis. Water and electrolytes, especially sodium and potassium are lost in the stools. The loss of bicarbonate ion from the stool may give rise to metabolic acidosis. Convulsions in children with gastroenteritis may be febrile, or less commonly due to hypernatraemia or cerebral vein thrombosis.

40 **A** = False **B** = True **C** = True **D** = True **E** = True

Chickenpox has an incubation period of 2 to 3 weeks. If the mother contracts chickenpox within a week before delivery, the baby may have a severe disease with pneumonitis which may be fatal. Zoster immune globulin and acyclovir should be given. They may also be given to immunocompromised children who are infected with chickenpox. If a child is infected with chickenpox, there are often vesicles on the mucous membrane inside the mouth. Reye's syndrome is a rare complication of chickenpox.

41 **A** = True **B** = True **C** = True **D** = False **E** = False

Plagiocephaly is an asymmetrical abnormality of skull shape which is usually postural (due to intrauterine factors or nursing position), or uncommonly due to craniosynostosis (premature fusion of skull bones) or sternomastoid tumour. The most important cause to exclude is craniosynostosis, as surgery may be required. Premature fusion of a coronal suture tends to cause frontal plagiocephaly while occipital plagiocephaly or a parallelogram-shaped skull is usually postural in origin.

42 **A** = False **B** = False **C** = False **D** = True **E** = True

School refusal often occurs when the child starts school, and during transition between primary and secondary school at 11 years of age. The child often complains of abdominal pain or headache, or simply refuses to go to school, and stays at home. The child is usually conscientious with a good academic record. On the other hand, truancy usually occurs later. Children leave home, but never arrive at school. Parents are often unaware that they are not attending school. They may have antisocial behaviour.

43 **A** = False **B** = True **C** = False **D** = True **E** = True

Haemorrhagic disease of the newborn presents between the second and fifth day of life and occurs mainly in breast-fed babies because of the inadequate vitamin K content of breast milk. Symptoms include bleeding from the umbilical stump, haematemesis, melaena and oozing from puncture sites. CNS bleeding occurs rarely, but pulmonary haemorrhage is not a feature. The incidence has been very greatly reduced by administration of vitamin K at birth.

44 **A** = False **B** = True **C** = False **D** = False **E** = False

Although ostium secundum atrial septal defects can occur in Trisomy 21, the more common defects are ventricular septal defects and ostium primum defects. Ostium secundum defects are usually asymptomatic, and present with a systolic murmur which is due to increased flow through the pulmonary valve. Fixed splitting of the second heart sound is heard. The defect is rarely, if ever, complicated by bacterial endocarditis.

45 **A** = True **B** = True **C** = False **D** = False **E** = True

Macroglossia occurs in babies with hypothyroidism, which should be rarely seen because of neonatal screening. Beckwith–Wiedemann's syndrome consists of macroglossia, macrosomia, exomphalos and neonatal hypoglycaemia. The cause of a protruding tongue in babies with Down's syndrome is a small mouth rather than a large tongue.

46 A = False **B** = True **C** = False **D** = True **E** = True

Turner's syndrome is associated with coarctation of the aorta, while Noonan's syndrome is associated with pulmonary stenosis. Congenital heart defects occur in about 40% of children with Down's syndrome, most commonly ventricular septal defect and endocardial cushion defects. Cardiac rhabdomyomata are probably quite common in infants with tuberous sclerosis and may cause arrhythmia and cardiac failure but the lesions may regress with time. Mitral regurgitation is common in Marfan's syndrome but the most serious defect is dilatation of the ascending aorta with the risk of catastrophic aortic dissection.

47 A = False **B** = True **C** = False **D** = True **E** = True

Homozygous beta thalassaemia may be diagnosed prenatally by DNA analysis of a chorionic villous biopsy specimen after 10 weeks gestation. If affected, the child is not anaemic at birth, but the haemoglobin falls progressively during the first few months of life. Some children with homozygous beta thalassaemia may maintain a haemoglobin between 7 g/dl and 10 g/dl. These children have thalassaemia intermedia and may not require regular transfusion if their growth is satisfactory and they do not develop skeletal changes. Iron overload, the major problem in transfusion-dependent thalassaemia patients results in endocrine complications, e.g. delayed puberty, diabetes and hypothyroidism. Bone marrow transplantation, if a suitable HLA compatible donor can be found, has resulted in long-term cure with good survival figures.

48 A = False **B** = True **C** = True **D** = True **E** = False

Syncope or fainting rarely happens without preceding symptoms such as nausea or light-headedness. The patient has marked pallor and a weak or impalpable pulse. Syncope may terminate with brief muscle jerking and urinary incontinence probably due to cerebral anoxia. Anticonvulsants are ineffective and contraindicated in syncope.

49 A = False **B** = False **C** = True **D** = False **E** = True

Absence attacks usually begin between 5 and 12 years and are more common in girls. They are rarely associated with learning difficulties or structural brain abnormalities. Sodium valproate or ethosuximide are the most effective anticonvulsant drugs. The prognosis is good although some children develop tonic-clonic seizures later.

50 A = False **B** = True **C** = True **D** = True **E** = False

Specific reading disorder is a specific and significant impairment of the development of reading skills, which is not totally accounted for by low mental age, poor vision, or inadequate schooling. Affected children often have associated slow oral reading speed and poor oral reading skills, poor reading comprehension, and spelling difficulties.

51 **A** = False **B** = False **C** = True **D** = True **E** = False

Von Willebrand's disease, Huntington's chorea and achondroplasia all have autosomal dominant inheritance.

52 **A** = False **B** = True **C** = True **D** = False **E** = True

Plagiocephaly is usually a benign condition associated with a strong head preference to one side and not with underlying intracranial pathology. Other mild asymmetries may occur (e.g. thoracic asymmetry). The condition becomes less obvious as the child becomes ambulant. However, in severely handicapped children postural asymmetry may persist and worsen with increasing age.

53 **A** = False **B** = True **C** = True **D** = True **E** = False

Most of the commonly used anticonvulsants have been implicated as teratogens. Craniofacial and digital abnormalities occur in 10% of fetuses exposed to phenytoin and the incidence of microcephaly, facial clefts and congenital heart disease is increased. Exposure *in utero* to sodium valproate has been associated with spina bifida as well as other congenital abnormalities. Warfarin exposure *in utero* is associated with craniofacial abnormalities and skeletal abnormalities.

54 **A** = False **B** = True **C** = True **D** = False **E** = False

Cystic fibrosis which affects 1 child in every 2000 can be diagnosed in early pregnancy by chorionic villous biopsy following identification of the cystic fibrosis gene in 1989. Although meconium ileus, chest infection and malabsorption are the main presentations, the condition may also present with liver problems, rectal prolapse, nasal polyposis, poor growth and male infertility. For the sweat test to be reliable, 100 mg sweat is necessary. For diagnosis, three sweat tests should be abnormal. A diet high in protein and calories is necessary and fat should never be restricted.

55 **A** = False **B** = False **C** = True **D** = False **E** = True

Sixty per cent of sudden infant death syndrome cases occur in the six winter months. The incidence is significantly less in Asian families and in babies who sleep in the supine position. Smoking during and after pregnancy and over-wrapping are significant risk factors. The incidence is also increased in mothers who are less than 20 years of age, in social classes IV and V, if the inter-pregnancy interval is short, in low birth weight babies, in twins and in boys.

56 **A** = False **B** = False **C** = True **D** = True **E** = False

The 21-hydroxylase deficiency accounts for 90% of cases of congenital adrenal hyperplasia and may present as ambiguous genitalia in females. Genitalia usually appear normal in males at birth who may present with a salt losing crisis towards the end of the first week or with precocious puberty later if they are not salt losers. A few late onset cases may present with delayed menarche, hirsutism and infertility. Hypertension is a feature of other enzyme defects such as 11-beta hydroxylase deficiency.

57 **A** = False **B** = False **C** = False **D** = True **E** = False

Fetal haemoglobin which consists of 2 alpha and 2 gamma chains comprises about 75% of total haemoglobin at birth and has a higher affinity for oxygen than adult haemoglobin. Fetal haemoglobin declines more slowly in children with beta thalassaemia and sickle cell disease and continues to be elevated throughout life.

58 **A** = True **B** = False **C** = True **D** = False **E** = True

Most children cannot stand on one leg for 10 seconds until the age of 5. A 3-year old child will usually draw a man with head and usually one or two other parts of the body.

59 **A** = True **B** = False **C** = False **D** = True **E** = True

Young infants with pertussis may present with apnoeic episodes or pneumonia. Children are most infectious during the catarrhal phase which precedes the onset of paroxysmal coughing. Fever is uncommon and would suggest possible secondary bacterial infection. In the convalescent phase, coughing and vomiting may persist for weeks to months.

60 **A** = True **B** = True **C** = True **D** = False **E** = True

In the United Kingdom, acquired hypothyroidism is most often due to autoimmune thyroiditis, although, wordwide, iodine deficiency is probably a commoner cause. The physical signs of hypothyroidism are often sparse and short stature is the most obvious symptom. Thyrotrophin releasing hormone (TRH) stimulates prolactin and follicle stimulating hormone (FSH) which may result in breast enlargement in girls. Boys may have enlarged testes. Although affected children may be quiet and placid, mental handicap does not occur. Hypothyroidism is commoner in children with Down's syndrome and also Turner's and Noonan's syndromes.

INDEX

Note: This index has been designed so that the user can identify the type of test(s) in which a topic is covered.
The first number in parentheses after each entry is that of the test. This is followed by the number of the multiple choice question (number only), the case commentary number (CC followed by number) or the short note question number (SN followed by number). Numbers outside parentheses are page numbers.